Pain Management

Editors

STEPHEN D. KRAU
MARIA OVERSTREET

CRITICAL CARE NURSING CLINICS OF NORTH AMERICA

www.ccnursing.theclinics.com

Consulting Editor
JAN FOSTER

December 2017 • Volume 29 • Number 4

ELSEVIER

1600 John F. Kennedy Boulevard • Suite 1800 • Philadelphia, Pennsylvania, 19103-2899

http://www.theclinics.com

CRITICAL CARE NURSING CLINICS OF NORTH AMERICA Volume 29, Number 4
December 2017 ISSN 0899-5885, ISBN-13: 978-0-323-55272-1

Editor: Kerry Holland
Developmental Editor: Laura Fisher

Critical Care Nursing Clinics of North America (ISSN 0899-5885) is published quarterly by Elsevier Inc., 360 Park Avenue South, New York, NY 10010-1710. Months of issue are March, June, September, and December. Business and Editorial Offices: 1600 John F. Kennedy Blvd., Suite 1800, Philadelphia, PA 19103-2899. Periodicals postage paid at New York, NY and additional mailing offices. Subscription prices are $155.00 per year for US individuals, $385.00 per year for US institutions, $100.00 per year for US students and residents, $200.00 per year for Canadian individuals, $483.00 per year for Canadian institutions, $230.00 per year for international individuals, $483.00 per year for international institutions and $115.00 per year for Canadian and international students/residents. To receive student/resident rate, orders must be accompanied by name of affiliated institution, data of term, and the *signature* of program/residency coordinator on institution letterhead. Orders will be billed at individual rate until proof of status is received. Foreign air speed delivery is included in all *Clinics* subscription prices. All prices are subject to change without notice. **POSTMASTER:** Send address changes to *Critical Care Nursing Clinics of North America*, Elsevier Health Sciences Division, Subscription Customer Service, 3251 Riverport Lane, Maryland Heights, MO 63043. **Customer Service: 1-800-654-2452 (US and Canada); 314-447-8871 (outside US and Canada). Fax: 314-447-8029. E-mail:** JournalsCustomerService-usa@elsevier.com **(for print support) and** JournalsOnlineSupport-usa@elsevier.com **(for online support).**

Reprints. For copies of 100 or more of articles in this publication, please contact the Commercial Reprints Department, Elsevier Inc., 360 Park Avenue South, New York, New York, 10010-1710; Tel.: 212-633-3874, Fax: 212-633-3820, and E-mail: reprints@elsevier.com.

Critical Care Nursing Clinics of North America is covered in *MEDLINE/PubMed (Index Medicus), International Nursing Index, Nursing Citation Index, Cumulative Index to Nursing and Allied Health Literature,* and *RNdex Top 100.*

Contributors

CONSULTING EDITOR

JAN FOSTER, PhD, APRN, CNS
Formerly, Associate Professor, College of Nursing, Texas Woman's University, Houston, Texas; Currently, President, Nursing Inquiry and Intervention, Inc, The Woodlands, Texas

EDITORS

STEPHEN D. KRAU, PhD, RN, CNE
Associate Professor, Vanderbilt University School of Nursing, Vanderbilt University, Nashville, Tennessee

MARIA OVERSTREET, PhD, RN
Dean, Nurse Anesthesia, Middle Tennessee School of Anesthesia, Madison, Tennessee

AUTHORS

ALISON R. ANDERSON, MSN, NP-C, ANP-BC
Vanderbilt University School of Nursing, Vanderbilt University, Nashville, Tennessee

BRYAN ANDERSON, DNAP, CRNA
Middle Tennessee School of Anesthesia, Madison, Tennessee

ROBERT S. ANTHONY, BS
Vanderbilt University School of Nursing, Vanderbilt University, Nashville, Tennessee

SEBASTIAN A. ATALLA, BS
Vanderbilt University School of Nursing, Vanderbilt University, Nashville, Tennessee

AMY CONNER BLACK, MSN, APRN, FNP-C
Assistant Professor, School of Nursing, Austin Peay State University, Clarksville, Tennessee

TONY BURCH, DNAP, CRNA
Murfreesboro, Tennessee

MARGARET L. CAMPBELL, PhD, RN, FPCN
Professor, College of Nursing, Wayne State University, Detroit, Michigan

MICHELLE R. COLLINS, PhD, CNM, FACNM, FAAN
Director, Nurse-Midwifery Program, University Nurse-Midwifery Practice, Professor, Vanderbilt University School of Nursing, Vanderbilt University, Nashville, Tennessee

NINA COYLE, BSPH
Nashville, Tennessee

LINDA DARNELL, MSN, RN
Associate Professor, School of Nursing, Austin Peay State University, Clarksville, Tennessee

OZZIE DeJESUS, DNAP, CRNA
Professor, Wolford College, Naples, Florida

JIE DENG, PhD, RN, OCN, FAAN
Vanderbilt University School of Nursing, Vanderbilt University, Nashville, Tennessee

DEBORAH L. ELLISON, PhD, MSN
Professor, School of Nursing, Austin Peay State University, Clarksville, Tennessee

FRANCISCA CISNEROS FARRAR, EdD, MSN, RN
Professor, School of Nursing, Austin Peay State University, Clarksville, Tennessee

AMY S. HAMLIN, PhD, MSN, FNP-BC, APRN
Professor, School of Nursing, Austin Peay State University, Clarksville, Tennessee

JENNIFER G. HENSLEY, EdD, CNM, WHNP, LCCE
Faculty, School of Nursing, The University of Texas at Austin, Austin, Texas

CLAIRE L. LEEZER, MSN, CNM
Faculty, Nurse-Midwifery Program, University Nurse-Midwifery Practice, Instructor, Vanderbilt University School of Nursing, Vanderbilt University, Nashville, Tennessee

TODD B. MONROE, PhD, RN-BC, FNAP, FGSA, FAAN
Vanderbilt University School of Nursing, Department of Psychiatry and Behavioral Health, Vanderbilt University School of Medicine, Vanderbilt University, Nashville, Tennessee

PATTY MONTGOMERY ORR, EdD, MSN, RN
Professor, School of Nursing, Austin Peay State University, Clarksville, Tennessee

KERI H. ORTEGA, DNAP, CRNA
Assistant Program Director, Wolford College, Naples, Florida

T. MICHELLE ROBERTSON, DNP, FNP-BC, APRN
Professor, School of Nursing, Austin Peay State University, Clarksville, Tennessee

SCOTT J. SEIPEL, PhD
Associate Professor, Department of Computer Information Systems, Jones College of Business, Middle Tennessee State University, Murfreesboro, Tennessee

BETTINA COBB SHANK, MSN, BSN, RN
Assistant Professor, School of Nursing, Austin Peay State University, Clarksville, Tennessee

MICHELE ANN WALTERS, DNP, APRN, FNP-BC, CNE
Associate Professor of Nursing, Department of Nursing, Morehead State University, Family Nurse Practitioner, St. Claire Regional Family Medicine, Morehead, Kentucky

DANIELLE WHITE, MSN, RN
Associate Professor, School of Nursing, Austin Peay State University, Clarksville, Tennessee

Contents

Acutely ill patients are challenging to frontline nurses because they frequently also have multiple chronic conditions. This article empowers all nurses to develop a foundational understanding of the physiology of acute and chronic pain. The skills, knowledge, and attitude to care for patients experiencing pain are a legal and ethical responsibility of all nurses. This article discusses the physiology of pain to include the neuronal receptors that respond to various painful stimuli, substances that stimulate nociceptors, the nerve pathways, modulation of the perception of pain, and acute verses chronic physiologic changes.

Pain is a multidimensional experience that can significantly impair an individual's quality of life. This article describes the pain classification systems, including anatomic, etiologic, intensity, duration, pathophysiological, and conditions that are not easily classified. A holistic approach is taken by addressing key components to assist with effective pain management, including the psychological and spiritual aspects of care. A case study scenario demonstrates the implementation of pain classifications in pain management. Also discussed are current controversies, potential genetic impacts, and the barriers chronic pain sufferers face, including addiction, diversion, and socioeconomic factors.

Patient satisfaction is evolving into an important measure of high-quality health care and anesthesia care is no exception. Pain management is an integral part of anesthesia care and must be assessed to determine patient satisfaction; therefore, it is a measure for quality of care. One issue is how patients reflect individual experiences into their overall anesthesia experience. There is a need to identify how postoperative pain scores correlate with anesthesia patient satisfaction survey results. Postoperative pain is not a dominant measure in determining anesthesia patient satisfaction.

Serious life-threatening respiratory depression may occur with pharmacologic pain intervention. The nurse has an ethical and legal duty to provide safe, quality, and accountable pain management. The nurse must acquire self-efficacy for the administration of pain medications for critically ill patients to prevent serious side effects and adverse reactions. This article presents a clinical toolkit for acute pain pharmacologic management by presenting professional guidelines, evidence-based pain assessment tools, common pain medication therapy, and focused monitoring specific to the drug. Medical adjustments owing to special populations is also discussed. Case reports demonstrate application of clinical reasoning skills needed for pain management.

Treatment of both acute and chronic pain typically involves a combination of pharmacologic and provider-based interventions, which is effective for some patients but not for others. Use of pain medications, especially repeated and frequent usage, involves the risk of adverse reactions, overuse, and dependency. Complementary and alternative therapies (CAT) offer an alternative or adjunctive method to decrease the pain experience and enhance function and quality of life. Various evidence-based CAT methods have been proved to be effective in the management of both acute and chronic pain. Nurses are well placed to implement various CAT modalities.

Dyspnea is a subjective experience of breathing discomfort that can be known only through a patient's report. Numeric rating or visual analog scales allow assessment of intensity when the patient can self-report. The Respiratory Distress Observation Scale is a valid, reliable tool for estimating distress when self-report cannot be elicited. Treating dyspnea begins with managing the underlying condition. Other dyspnea-specific evidence-based interventions include morphine and fentanyl, upright positioning, oxygen, invasive and noninvasive ventilation, and balancing rest with activity. Effectiveness has not been established for benzodiazepines, nebulized furosemide, oxygen in the face of normoxemia, other opioids, and nebulized fentanyl.

Critical care clinicians may be called on to care for a laboring woman. Comprehension of the anatomic changes associated with pregnancy, and labor and birth, is essential. A working knowledge of the current options for pain management in labor, both pharmacologic and nonpharmacologic, is necessary to facilitate patient-centered care. Pharmacologic options include intravenous or intramuscular agents, inhalational agents, and neuraxial anesthesia. Each modality has contraindications, risks, and benefits that must be considered when choosing the most appropriate method.

Chronic stable angina (CSA) is a symptomatic problem that is precipitated by ischemic heart disease. CSA is diagnosed when symptoms are present for at least 2 months without changes in severity, character, or triggering circumstances. This article is a summary of current treatment strategies aimed to prevent progression of atherosclerosis, and medication therapies to control angina symptoms and improve quality of life for the individual.

Pain control in parturients can be particularly challenging for the hospital staff. To achieve optimal outcomes in anesthesia patients, it is important to consider multiple options for pain control, especially when traditional options pose a problem or are not options. In particular, there are parturient clients for whom the use of neuraxial anesthesia (epidural and spinal blockade) is not an option. One option that warrants consideration for patient-centered anesthesia practice is the use of remifentanil.

The risk of pain in adults with dementia worsens with advancing age. Painful comorbidities may be underassessed and inadequately treated. Receiving treatment in critical care settings may indicate greater occurrences of pain and complications. Pain may exacerbate behavioral and psychological symptoms of dementia (BPSD), such as agitation. Complementary and alternative medicine therapies may alleviate pain and BPSD, and continuity of therapy may bolster these therapeutic effects. This article did not reveal an apparent benefit of aromatherapy; however, improvements in BPSD have been shown previously. Massage and human interaction did demonstrate efficacy in reducing BPSD and pain.

CRITICAL CARE NURSING CLINICS OF NORTH AMERICA

Preface

Pain Today

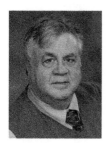 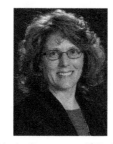

Stephen D. Krau, PhD, RN, CNE   Maria Overstreet, PhD, RN
Editors

Daily, news headlines list the number of deaths from an opioid crisis plaguing Americans without regard to age, gender, race, economic status, or acute and chronic disease states. Acute and critical care nurses face daily the patients and families affected by this crisis as well as those who receive their first opioid dose while in the hospital. Can we as nurses make a difference in this crisis by changing our daily practice? Yes, we can. We encourage each nurse to learn more about the theories of pain, the physiology of pain, as well as current evidenced-based treatments of pain in your specialty of practice. Then, we challenge you to begin the dialogue with your colleagues to rethink how as nurses we can offer safer and more effective options for pain control to our patients.

The inspiration for this issue came about while we worked together to assist in the creation of a robust curriculum plan for an Acute Surgical Pain Management Fellowship for Certified Registered Nurse Anesthetists. We discussed how the concept of pain, assessment, and management of pain has changed over the years. We have witnessed in our own practice how the concept of pain has moved on a continuum from expected patient pain postsurgically to a patient-centered experience of pain, meaning, pain is what the patient states it is.

This issue of *Critical Care Nursing Clinics of North America* focuses on pain. The articles address a variety of topics related to pain, including the physiology of pain, classifications, assessment, and interventions for pain. More specifically, it addresses pain in regards to illness and health in the respiratory system, obstetrics, and with chronic cardiac angina. Two articles, in particular, arose from doctoral and postdoctoral work and focus on particular treatments of pain: the intricate use of an agent for analgesia and complementary and alternative treatment of pain for patients with dementia in long-term care facilities.

Providing quality care includes the assessment and management of the patients' pain experience. The treatment of pain, or better yet, the attempt to make the

Crit Care Nurs Clin N Am 29 (2017) ix–x
http://dx.doi.org/10.1016/j.cnc.2017.09.001
0899-5885/17/© 2017 Published by Elsevier Inc.

experience of pain less intense and manageable for patients, has also changed over the years. Acute and critical care nurses have a responsibility of performing a quick and thorough assessment, providing evidenced-based interventions and evaluation of effect. Nurses also have the responsibility of life-long learning. This collection of articles will challenge nurses to reevaluate their knowledge level of pain as well as gain an appreciation for alternative therapies to share with their colleagues.

Stephen D. Krau, PhD, RN, CNE
Vanderbilt School of Nursing
380 Frist Hall
461 21st Avenue South
Nashville, TN 37240, USA

Maria Overstreet, PhD, RN
Middle Tennessee School of Anesthesia
315 Hospital Drive
Madison, TN 37116, USA

E-mail addresses:
Steve.Krau@vanderbilt.edu (S.D. Krau)
m.overstreet@mtsa.edu (M. Overstreet)

Physiology of Pain

Deborah L. Ellison, PhD, MSN

KEYWORDS

• Physiology of pain • Nociception • Neuropathic • Acute pain • Chronic pain

KEY POINTS

- Nociception involves the normal functioning of physiologic systems, which encompasses four stages: transduction, transmission, perception, and modulation.
- The patients' pain threshold and tolerance are subjective and influence an individual's perception of pain.
- The perception of pain can therefore be influenced by genetics, gender, cultural perceptions, expectations, role socialization, physical and mental health, past pain, and age.
- Pain is one the body's most important, adaptive, and protective mechanisms.

INTRODUCTION

Assessing pain in the critical care unit (CCU) is challenging for the frontline nurse. Regardless of patient diagnosis, all patients in the CCU share a common complaint of pain. Although many patients in the CCU can self-report pain, there are also many patients in this setting that have difficulty communicating because of a variety of reasons, such as mechanical intubation, high-dose sedation, level of consciousness, neuromuscular blocking agents, and language or cultural barriers.[1] Effective pain management results in improved patient outcomes and increased patient satisfaction if delivered with an individualized, balanced approach, using interdisciplinary methods.[2] The frontline nurse can improve pain assessments and interventions by first understanding the physiology of pain, while practicing safe quality patient-centered care. This article discusses the physiology of pain to include the neuronal receptors that respond to various painful stimuli, substances that stimulate nociceptors, the nerve pathways, modulation of the perception of pain, and acute verses chronic physiologic changes.

SCOPE OF PROBLEM

The International Association for the Study of Pain defines pain as "an unpleasant sensory emotional experience with actual or potential tissue damage, or describe in terms

Disclosure Statement: The author does not have any commercial or financial conflicts of interest and any funding sources.
School of Nursing, Austin Peay State University, 601 College Street, Clarksville, TN 37043, USA
E-mail address: ellisond@apsu.edu

of such damage."[3] This definition is accepted universally and by the American Nurses Association.[2] Pain is difficult to define because of the subjective nature of self-reporting, which encompasses sensory, emotional, cognitive, and social components.[4]

Assessing and treating pain is a responsibility of all nurses in all health care settings. Nurses have a legal and ethical responsibility to have the knowledge, skills, and attitude to provide the best pain care possible. Nevertheless, with more than 100 million Americans suffering from chronic pain,[5,6] this complicates the pain assessment in the CCU setting because nurses are confronted with patients with acute pain and life-threatening issues. How pain is transmitted and perceived is complex because of the level of subjectivity in reporting and because of the nature of the fully integrated constantly changing structure of the central nervous system, the symphony of chemical mediators. Most CCU patients experience pain while in the CCU setting and concerns about having pain during the stay certainly add stress to patients. Patients expect and have a right to receive adequate pain relief.[7] **Table 1** outlines the physiologic impact of pain, the impact on quality of life, and the financial impact of unrelieved pain.

NOCICEPTION

Nociception is the term that is used to describe how pain becomes a conscious experience.[8] Nociception involves the normal functioning of physiologic systems. A nociceptor is a free nerve ending (dendrites) preferentially sensitive to a noxious stimulus or to a stimulus that would become noxious if prolonged. Nociceptors are a highly specialized subset of primary sensory neurons that respond only to pain stimuli[9] and convert the stimuli into nerve impulses, which the brain interprets to produce the sensation of pain.[10] Nociceptors are categorized either as myelinated or unmyelinated, which indicates the kind of stimulation they respond to: chemical, mechanical, and thermal stimuli.[9,11,12] There are four phases in the nociception of pain: (1) transduction, (2) transmission, (3) perception, and (4) modulation (**Fig. 1**).

Transduction is the first process of nociception. Transduction refers to the conversion of a noxious stimulus (thermal, mechanical, or chemical) into electrical activity in the peripheral terminals of nociceptor sensory fibers.[9] This first process begins when

Table 1 Impact of unrelieved pain		
Physiologic Impact	**Quality of Life Impact**	**Financial Impact**
• Prolongs stress response • Increases heart rate, blood pressure, and oxygen demand • Decreases gastrointestinal motility • Causes immobility • Decreases immune response • Delays healing • Poorly managed acute pain increases risk for development of chronic pain	• Interferes with activities of daily living • Causes anxiety, depression, hopelessness, fear, anger, and sleeplessness • Impairs family, work, and social relationships	• Costs Americans billions of dollars per year • Increases hospital length of stay • Leads to loss of income and productivity

Data from Refs.[4,8,13]

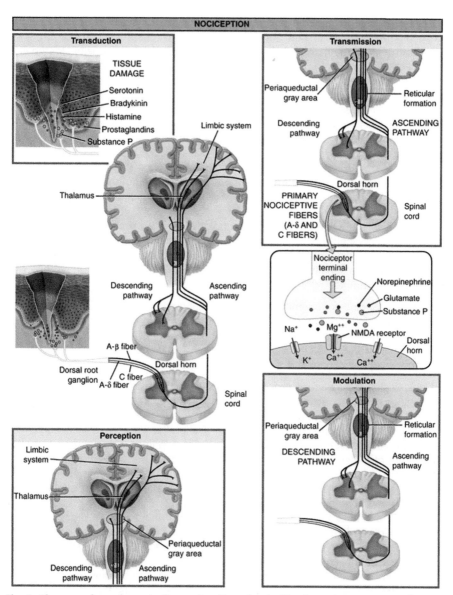

Fig. 1. There are four phases in the nociception of pain. The four phases are transduction, transmission, perception, and modulation. (*From* Ignatavicius D, Workman ML. Assessment and care of patients with pain. Medical-surgical nursing: patient-centered collaborative care. 8th edition. St Louis (MO): Elsevier; 2016. p. 24–49.)

nociceptors are activated by a noxious stimulus, causing ion channel (sodium, potassium, calcium) on the nociceptors to open, creating electrical impulses that travel through axons of two primary types of nociceptors that are transmitted to the spinal cord, brainstem, thalamus, and cortex.[9,11,13] There are two primary types of nociceptors: A delta fibers and C fibers.

The A delta are myelinated nociceptors that are large, fast-conducting fibers.[8,9] Some respond readily to heat (eg, mechanothermal receptors in a burn); others are high-threshold mechanoreceptors. The A delta fibers are responsible for the first or immediate sharp pain.[9] Activation of these fibers causes a spinal reflex withdrawal of the affected body part from the stimulus, before a pain sensation is perceived.

The C fibers are smaller unmyelinated fibers that constitute most peripheral nociceptors.[9] The C fibers are located in muscles tendons, body organs, and the skin.[12] They transmit dull, aching, or burning sensations that are poorly localized and often present as a constant pain. Most C fibers are classified as C-polymodal nociceptors because they respond to thermal, mechanical, and chemical stimuli.[9] These are slow-conducting and recover from fatigue more slowly than those of A delta nociceptors. C fibers produce longer-lasting pain, typically characterized as a dull pain.[9,12]

The nociceptors when stimulated directly release several chemicals that further activate more nociceptors.[8] The chemicals that increase transmission of pain include histamine, bradykinin, acetylcholine, serotonin, and substance P.[1] These chemicals can either increase sensitivity of pain or reduce or inhibit the perception of pain. The following are examples[12,14]:

- Prostaglandins are chemical substances that are believed to increase the sensitivity of pain receptors by enhancing the pain-provoking effect of bradykinin
- Substance P is a chemical found in C fibers and amplifies the pain signal
- Chemicals that inhibit the transmission or perception of pain, such as endorphins and enkephalins, which is a natural opioid

Transmission is the second process involved in nociception. Transmission refers to the passage of action potentials from the peripheral terminal along axons to the central terminal of nociceptors in the central nervous system.[9,11] Conduction is the synaptic transfer of input from one neuron to another.[9] During this process, the conduction of pain impulses runs along both the A delta and C fibers (primary order neurons) into the dorsal horn of the spinal cord. Here they form synapses with excitatory or inhibitory interneurons (second order neurons) in the substantia gelatinosa of the dorsal horn.[9,11] It is during this time that pain control can take place. Opioids block the release of neurotransmitters, particularly substance P, which stops the pain at the spinal level. The impulses then synapse with projection neurons (third order neurons), cross the midline of the spinal cord, and ascend to the brain through two different spinothalamic tracts.[12,14] One tract, neospinothalamic tract, carries fast impulses for acute sharp pain. The paleospinothalamic tract carries slow impulses for dull or chronic pain. The fast sharp pain is perceived first, followed by dull, throbbing pain. These tracts connect to the reticular formation, hypothalamus, thalamus (the major relay station of sensory information), and limbic system.[12,14] The impulses are then projected to the somatosensory cortex for interpretation and to other areas of the brain for an integrated response to the pain stimuli.[12,14]

Perception is the third process involved in nociception. Perception refers to the "decoding"/interpretation of afferent input in the brain that gives rise to the individual's specific sensory experience.[9] This is the conscious awareness of pain. The transmission of the stimuli ends at in the reticular and limbic systems and the cerebral cortex, which is where the perception occurs.[9,12] This happens almost simultaneously. Interpretation of pain may be influenced by many factors, including but not limited to genetics, cultural preferences, gender roles, life experience, past pain experiences, and level of health.

There are three systems that interact to produce the perception of pain[9]:

- The sensory-discriminative system is mediated by the somatosensory cortex and is responsible for identifying the presence, character, location, and intensity of pain.
- The affective-motivational system determines an individual's conditioned avoidance behaviors and emotional responses to pain. It is mediated through the reticular formation, limbic system, and brainstem.
- The cognitive-evaluative system overlies the individual's learned behavior concerning the experience of pain and therefore can modulate perception of pain. It is mediated through the cerebral cortex. The integration of these three systems is referred to as the "pain matrix."

A patient's pain threshold and tolerance are subjective and influence an individual's perception of pain. The perception of pain can therefore be influenced by genetics, gender, cultural perceptions, expectations, role socialization, physical and mental health, past pain, and age.

Modulation is the last process in nociception. Modulation refers to the alteration (eg, augmentation or suppression) of sensory input.[9] In this final step, modulation of the pain stimuli before pain perception is by either inhibition or enhancement through supraspinal influences arising from the pons, medulla, and midbrain.[14,15] Supraspinal inhibition leads to release of endogenous opiates that limit the release of neurotransmitters from the primary neuron and hyperpolarize the secondary neuron so it requires greater stimuli to reach its action potential.[14,15] Other chemical releases at the dorsal horn are norepinephrine and serotonin; both are inhibitory but their exact action remains unclear. Suprasprinal stimulation occurs by releasing additional neurotransmitters to enhance the stimuli progression from primary to secondary neurons.[15] Essentially, the interneuron can be influenced by descending pathways from the brain or ascending pathways from the spinal cord.[14] Depending on which pathway, augments what the individual cognitively receives. Examples of pain modulation include when a person experiences an obvious painful stimulation but does not feel any pain, such as when someone is able to walk on hot coals; the opposite effect is when someone has a paper cut and experiences extreme pain.

NEUROPATHIC PAIN

Neuropathic pain is chronic pain initiated or caused by a primary lesion or dysfunction in the nervous system and leads to long-term changes in pain pathway structures (neuroplasticity) and abnormal processing of sensory information.[9,16] There is amplification of pain without stimulation by injury or inflammation. Neuropathic pain is often described as burning, shooting, shock-like, or tingling. It is characterized by increased sensitivity to painful or nonpainful stimuli with hyperalgesia, allodynia (the induction of pain by normally nonpainful stimuli), and the development of spontaneous pain.[9,17] Neuropathic pain is classified as either peripheral or central and is associated with central and peripheral sensitization.[9,18] Neuropathic pain is unique because it cannot be described as either acute or chronic. This type of pain can occur within days, weeks, or months. Most often neuropathic pain is below the level of injury, most often in the legs, thighs, and toes, but cannot be ruled out in the upper body. The following are a few of the specific neuropathic pain issues that may be seen:

- Sympathetically mediated pain is pain arising from a peripheral nerve lesion and associated with autonomic changes. Examples include complex regional pain syndrome I and II. This can result from a major injury or a minor trauma.[19,20]

- Peripheral neuropathic pain is caused by peripheral nerve lesions, an increase in the sensitivity and excitability of primary sensory neurons, and cells in the dorsal root ganglion (peripheral sensitization). Examples include nerve entrapment, diabetic neuropathy, or chronic pancreatitis.[9,14]
- Central neuropathic pain is caused by a lesion or dysfunction in the brain or spinal cord.[9] A progressive repeated stimulation of group C neurons (wind-up) in the dorsal horn leads to increased sensitivity of central pain signaling neurons (central sensitization). This results in pathologic changes in the central nervous system that cause chronic pain.[21] Examples include brain or spinal cord trauma, tumors, vascular lesions, multiple sclerosis, Parkinson disease, postherpetic neuralgia, and phantom limb pain.[22,23]

The following mechanisms have been implicated in the cause of neuropathic pain:

- Changes in sensitivity of neurons—lower threshold with peripheral and central sensitization[8,9,12,17]
- Spontaneous impulses from regenerating peripheral nerves[8,9,12]
- Alterations in the dorsal root ganglion and spinothalamic tract in response to peripheral nerve injury[8,9,12,24]
- Loss of pain inhibition and stimulation of pain facilitation by excitatory neurotransmitters in the dorsal horn[8,9,12]
- Loss of descending inhibitory pain modulation[8,9,24]
- Hyperexcitable spinal interneurons stimulated by A beta fibers (nonpainful stimulation of pain)[8,9,12]
- Release of nociceptive inflammatory cytokines, chemokines, and growth factors by activated glial cells[8,9,12,23]
- Structural and functional alterations in brain processing[8,9,12,24]

Neuropathic pain is difficult to treat because of the complexity of the causes and requires a multimodal treatment regime (**Table 2**).

CHRONIC VERSUS ACUTE PHYSIOLOGIC CHANGES

Physiologic pain is experienced when an intact, properly functioning nervous system sends signals that tissue are damaged, requiring attention and proper care. The critical care nurse understands that there are several physiologic parameters that can be used to evaluate, measure, and quantify the pain stimulus. The parameters include heart rate, respiratory rate, blood pressure, O_2 arterial saturation, transcutaneous oxygen and carbonic dioxide pressures, vagal tone, palmar sweating, and intracranial pressure. Although there are usually physiologic and/or behavioral responses to pain the CCU nurse must remember that the absence of physiologic and behavioral responses does not mean the absence of pain.[8] There are several reasons why an individual would not have acute physiologic responses, such as the fact that the patient had lived with the chronic pain for so long. The absence of acute physiologic responses could lead to a nurse not providing an accurate assessment and treatment of a patient's pain. **Table 3** summarizes the differences in acute and chronic pain.

PAIN AND AGING POPULATION

By 2050, one in five Americans will be older than 65 years of age, with those older than 85 showing the greatest increase in numbers. The number of people living to 100 years of age is projected to grow at more than 20 times the rate of the total population by 2050.[25] The aging population is complicated when it comes to understanding,

Table 2
Physiologic sources of nociceptive pain and neuropathic pain for acute and chronic pain

Physiologic Structure	Characteristics of Pain	Sources of Acute Postoperative Pain	Sources of Chronic Pain Syndromes
Nociceptive pain (normal pain processing)			
Somatic pain			
Cutaneous or superficial: skin and subcutaneous tissues	Sharp, burning, pricking (well localized)	Incisional pain, pain at insertion sites of tubes and drains, wound complication, orthopedic procedures, skeletal muscle spasms, inflammation	Bony metastases, osteoarthritis and rheumatoid arthritis, low back pain, peripheral vascular diseases
Deep somatic: bone, muscle, blood vessels, connective tissues	Dull, aching, cramping (localized and diffuse)		
Visceral pain			
Organs and the linings of the body cavities	Poorly localized diffuse, deep cramping or splitting, sharp, stabbing	Chest tubes, abdominal tubes and drains, bladder distention or spasms, intestinal distention	Pancreatitis, liver metastases, colitis, appendicitis
Neuropathic pain (abnormal pain processing)			
Peripheral or central nervous system: nerve fibers, spinal cord, and higher central nervous system	Poorly localized shooting, burning, tingling, fiery, shock-like, sharp, painful numbness, pins and needles sensation	Phantom limb pain, postmastectomy pain, nerve compression	Human immunodeficiency virus–related pain, diabetic neuropathy, chemotherapy-induced neuropathies, cancer-related nerve injury, radiculopathies

Data from Refs.[8,9,14,33]

assessing, and treatment of pain. Some older adults have an increase in pain threshold, whereas others have a decrease, often complaints may be vague and nonspecific, and atypical in presentation.[26] This may be caused by changes in peripheral neuropathies and changes in the thickness of skin.[10] Some older adults may become used to the constant pain and do not see the need in self-reporting. Some of the physiologic symptoms seen in the elderly include but are not limited to increased heart rate, blood pressure, and respiratory rate; flushing or pallor; sweating; nausea and vomiting; and decreased oxygen saturation.[10] The following information should be kept in mind when caring for the aging population in all health care settings:

- Studies on pain in older adults show that pain is prevalent but often underreported[27]
- 50% of adults 65 and older report they experienced pain in the last 30 days[27]
- Up to 80% of nursing home residents experience pain regularly without treatment or relief of pain[28]

Table 3
Summary of differences in acute and chronic pain

Acute Pain	Chronic Pain (or Persistent Pain)
• Results from noxious stimuli that activates nociceptors neuron.	• Results from nociceptors, visceral, or somatic.
• It accompanies surgery, traumatic injury, tissue damage, myocardial infarction, and inflammatory processes. Usually decreases when healing begins.	• It accompanies chronic disease, untreated condition. Usually begins gradually and persists inflecting more suffering over time.
• Self-limited, resolves over days to weeks, but can persist for up to 3 mo.	• Unresolved as long as underlying cause is present. Usually lasts longer than 3 mo (often durations of >6 mo)
• Can range from mild to severe.	• Can range from mild to severe.
• May be accompanied by anxiety and restlessness.	• Often accompanied by multiple quality-of-life and functional adverse effects including: depression; hopelessness; helplessness; fatigue; financial burden; and increased dependence on family, friends, and the health care system.
• When unrelieved, can increase morbidity and mortality and prolong hospital stay.	• Can impact the quality-of-life of family members and friends.
• If poorly managed can inhibit participation in recovery and subsequent increase in disability.	• Physiologic responses depend on whether persistent or intermittent. Intermittent pain physiologic response similar to that of acute pain includes tachycardia, diaphoresis, and elevated blood pressure.

Data from Refs.[8,10,14]

- More than 80% of older adults have chronic medical conditions that are typically associated with pain, such as osteoarthritis and peripheral vascular disease[29]
- Older adults often have multiple medical conditions, both acute and/or chronic, and may suffer from multiple types and sources of pain[29]
- Pain may be overreported to seek attention from family, and lack of reporting caused by a fear of being labeled as a complainer[30]

The aging population is rapidly growing and accounts for 46% of critical care patients and 60% of medical-surgical patients in the hospital.[25] These vulnerable and complex older adults require the development of specific gerontologic and pain knowledge and assessment skills to meet their unique needs.

SUMMARY

Pain is one the body's most important, adaptive, and protective mechanisms.[11,12,14] Unfortunately the physiology of pain perception is poorly understood but nurses must accept the legal and ethical issues that arise when caring for patients in pain and in all health care settings. Pain is commonly classified as nociceptive or neuropathic pain. Nociceptive originates in damaged tissues outside of the nervous system, including somatic and visceral pain. Neuropathic pain arises from abnormal neural activity and is classified as sympathetically medicated, peripheral, or central pain. Nurses must understand the basic physiology to provide effective pain management for acute and chronic pain across the continuum of care.

Acutely ill patients are challenging to frontline nurses because they frequently also have multiple chronic conditions. This article empowers all nurses to develop a foundational understanding of the physiology of acute and chronic pain. This allows for improvement in patient-centered care and patient outcomes. The skills, knowledge, and attitude to care for patients experiencing pain are a legal and ethical responsibility of all nurses. A hierarchical approach assists frontline nurses caring for all patients, whereby multiple sources of information are integrated by the examiner, starting with patient report, and including reports from observers (proxy reporting of pain), observation of patient behavior, use of behavioral pain assessment tools, and search for potential causes of pain.[31,32]

REFERENCES

1. Hylén M, Akerman E, Alm-Roijer C, et al. Behavioral Pain Scale: translation, reliability, and validity in a Swedish context. Acta Anaesthesiol Scand 2016;60(6):821–8.
2. American Nurses Association. Pain management nursing: scope and standards of practice. 2nd edition. Silver Springs (MD): American Nurses Association; 2016. ISBN: 9781558106598.
3. International Association for the Study of Pain. Part III. Pain terms, a current list with definition and notes on usage. 1194. Available at: http://www.iasp-pain. org/Eduation/Content.aspx?. Accessed April 20, 2017.
4. Williams AC, Craig KD. Updating the definition of pain. Pain 2016;157(11): 2420–3.
5. Institute of Medicine. Relieving pain in America: a blueprint for transforming prevention, care, education, and research. Available at: http://www.iom.edu/Reports/ 2011/Relieving-Pain-in-America-A-Blueprint-for-Transforming-Prevention-Care-Education-Research.aspx. Accessed April 20, 2017.
6. Dzau VJ, Pizzo PA. Relieving pain in America: insights from an Institute of Medicine committee. JAMA 2014;312:1507.
7. Barr J, Fraser GL, Puntillo K, et al. Clinical practice guidelines for the management of pain, agitation, and delirium in patients in the intensive care unit. Crit Care Med 2013;41:263–306.
8. Ignatavicius D, Workman ML. Chapter 3 assessment and care of patients with pain. Medical-surgical nursing: patient-centered collaborative care. 8th edition. St Louis (MO): Elsevier; 2016. p. 24–49. ISBN 978-1-4557-7255-1 VitalBook file.
9. Rosenquist EWK, Aronson MD, Crowley M. Definition and pathogenesis of chronic pain. Uptodate; 2017.
10. Patel NB. Chapter 3 physiology of pain from guide to pain management in low-resources settings. International Association for the Study of Pain; 2010. p. 14–7.
11. McCleskey EW, Gold MS. Ion channels of nociception. Annu Rev Physiol 1999; 61:835. Uptodate.
12. Huether S, McCance K. Understanding pathophysiology. 6th edition. Mosby; 2016. p. 340–2.
13. Potenoy RK, Dhingra LK. Overview of cancer pain syndromes. Uptodate; 2017.
14. Capriotti T, Frizzell JP. Pathophysiology: introductory concepts and clinical perceptions. Chapter 6 Pain. Philadelphia: F. A. Davis Company; 2016. p. 93–113. ISBN-13: 978-0803615717.
15. Lome B. Acute pain and critically Ill trauma patient. Crit Care Nurs Q 2005;28(2): 200–7.
16. Woolf CJ. Dissecting out mechanisms responsible for peripheral neuropathic pain: implications for diagnosis and therapy. Life Sci 2004;74:2605.

17. Waxman SG, Dib-Hajj S, Cummins TR, et al. Sodium channels and pain. Proc Natl Acad Sci U S A 1999;96:7635.
18. Ueda H. Molecular mechanisms of neuropathic pain-phenotypic switch and initiation mechanisms. Pharmacol Ther 2006;109:57.
19. Bennett M. The LANSS Pain Scale: the Leeds assessment of neuropathic symptoms and signs. Pain 2001;92:147.
20. Stanton-Hicks M, Jänig W, Hassenbusch S, et al. Reflex sympathetic dystrophy: changing concepts and taxonomy. Pain 1995;63:127.
21. Woolf CJ, Shortland P, Coggeshall RE. Peripheral nerve injury triggers central sprouting of myelinated afferents. Nature 1992;355:75.
22. Woolf CJ, Salter MW. Neuronal plasticity: increasing the gain in pain. Science 2000;288:1765.
23. Ji RR, Kohno T, Moore KA, et al. Central sensitization and LTP: do pain and memory share similar mechanisms? Trends Neurosci 2003;26:696.
24. Fukuoka T, Kondo E, Dai Y, et al. Brain-derived neurotrophic factor increases in the uninjured dorsal root ganglion neurons in selective spinal nerve ligation model. J Neurosci 2001;21:4891.
25. Ellison D, White D, Farrar F. Aging population. Nurs Clin North Am 2015;50(1): 185–213.
26. Kendall JL, Moreira ME. Evaluation of the adult with abdominal pain in the emergency department. Uptodate; 2017.
27. National Center for Health Statistics. National Center for Health Statistics Report: Health, United States, 2006 Special Feature on Pain. 2006. Available at: http://www.cdc.gov/nchs/pressroom/06facts/hus06.htm. Accessed April 20, 2017.
28. Zanocchi M, Maero B, Nicola E, et al. Chronic pain in a sample of nursing home residents: prevalence, characteristics, influence on quality of life (QoL). Arch Gerontol Geriatr 2008;47:121–8.
29. Horgas AL, Yoon SL. Pain: nursing standard of practice protocol pain management in older adults. Available at: http://consultgerirn.org/topics/pain/want_to_know_moreUptodate. Accessed April 20, 2017.
30. Flaherty E. Pain assessment for older adults. In: Greenberg SA, editor. Hartford geriatric nursing: best practices in nursing care of older adults. Issue 7. New York: New York University, College of Nursing; 2012. Available at: www.ConsultGeriRN.org. Accessed April 20, 2017.
31. Chang VT. Approach to symptom assessment in palliative care. Uptodate; 2017.
32. Herr K, Coyne PJ, McCaffery M, et al. Pain assessment in the patient unable to self-report: position statement with clinical practice recommendations. Pain Manag Nurs 2011;12:230.
33. Cowen R, Stasiowska MK, Laycock H, et al. Assessing pain objectively: the use of physiological markers. Anaesthesia 2015;70:828–47.

The Role of Pain Classification Systems in Pain Management

Patty Montgomery Orr, EdD, MSN, RN, Bettina Cobb Shank, MSN, BSN, RN*,
Amy Conner Black, MSN, APRN, FNP-C

KEYWORDS

- Pain • Classification • Etiologic • Pathophysiological • Duration • Intensity
- Pain management • Pain assessment

KEY POINTS

- Pain classification systems are key evidenced-based methods of documentation that assist with formulating subjective and objective assessment data in pain management.
- Incorporating a holistic approach to pain management is essential to achieve desired patient outcomes.
- Health care professionals must be proactive and recognize potential negative consequences and barriers in pain management, including addiction, misuse, psychological aspects, genetic factors, and socioeconomic considerations.

INTRODUCTION

The International Association for the Study of Pain (IASP) defines pain as "an unpleasant sensory and emotional experience associated with actual or potential tissue damage, or described in terms of such damage."[1–3] Pain is a universal experience and continues to be the predominant reason for health care encounters.[4] The American Academy of Pain Medicine reports that pain touches more Americans than the chronic diseases of cancer, diabetes, and heart disease combined.[5] According to the Joint Commission International, Margo McCaffrey's definition of pain is the gold standard for patient treatment in clinical practice. McCaffrey defines pain as "whatever the experiencing person says it is, existing whenever he or she says it does."[1,3]

Disclosure Statement: Dr P.M. Orr, B.C. Shank and A.C. Black have no relationships with any commercial company and do not have any direct financial interest in the subject matter or materials discussed in the submitted article or with a company making a competing product.
School of Nursing, Austin Peay State University, 601 College Street, Clarksville, TN 37044, USA
* Corresponding author.
E-mail address: shankb@apsu.edu

RELEVANCE TO CLINICAL PRACTICE

Health care professionals strive to achieve effective pain management in clinical practice. Pain management can be a dynamically complex task with the primary goal of achieving satisfactory results for the patient's quality of life. Health care professionals are equipped with evidence-based practices and resources to assist in making sound clinical judgment. To start the pain assessment process, recognizing and understanding the value of pain classification systems in the clinical decision-making process is vital to providing appropriate care for each patient experiencing pain.

CLASSIFICATION SYSTEMS

Key classification systems synthesized in clinical practice include anatomic, etiologic, intensity, duration, and pathophysiological classifications. According to the World Health Organization (WHO), anatomic, etiologic, duration, and pathophysiological are the most commonly used classification systems.[2] A comprehensive approach is the optimal plan of action in effective pain management. Pain classification systems are 1-dimensional and the need to apply the systems using a multimodal approach is evident.[6]

Anatomic

The Anatomic Pain classification system describes the specific region or area of the body that is perceived to be experiencing pain. When applicable, it is often the first classification system used to identify the body location experiencing pain. The "Where is Your Pain" diagram is a useful tool to assist with assessment and documentation of pain.[7]

Etiologic

The Etiologic Pain classification system describes the causative factor of pain. Etiologic classification of pain can be subdivided into malignant versus nonmalignant to reference cancerous versus noncancerous causes of pain.[2,6] Etiologic pain factors include acute injury or underlying disease and/or condition. The underlying disease or condition can be acute or chronic in nature. It may be due to the treatment of the underlying disease or condition, including surgical interventions.[3]

Intensity

The Pain Intensity classification system can be measured through visual, numerical, rating, and/or descriptor scales.[7] The National Institute of Pain Control recognizes the Wong-Baker Faces Pain Scale, the 0 to 10 Numeric Pain Rating Scale, the Verbal Pain Intensity Scale, the Neuropathic Pain Scale, the Descriptor Differential Scale, and the Visual Analog Scale (**Fig. 1**).[7]

In *Pain Management Nursing Scope and Standards of Practice*, 2nd edition, the American Nurses Association (ANA) provides resources for pain assessment using intensity scales. The adult recommendations include the following:

For adolescents and adults
- Numeric Pain Rating Scale
- Verbal Descriptor Pain Scale
- FACES Pain Scale, revised
- Wong-Baker FACES Pain Rating Scale
- Iowa Pain Scale
- Functional Pain Scale

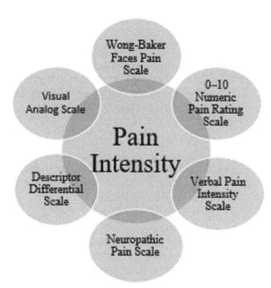

Fig. 1. Pain scales. (*Data from* the National Initiative on Pain Control. Pain assessment scales. Available at: https://www.painedu.org/downloads/nipc/pain%20assessment%20scales.pdf. Accessed March 9, 2017.)

- Critical Care Pain Observational Tool
- Brief Pain Inventory
- McGill Pain Assessment Tool

Nonverbal or cognitively impaired
- Adult Nonverbal Pain Scale
- Checklist of Nonverbal Pain Indicators
- Pain Assessment in Advanced Dementia Scale.[8]

Duration

The Duration of Pain classification system represents the duration of time the patient experiences pain. The 2 primary duration classifications are acute and chronic pain. The ANA recognizes duration as "Temporal Pattern," and further subdivides it into 3 categories: acute, chronic, and episodic.[8]

Acute pain represents short-term pain that resolves within a 3 to 6 months.[8] Acute pain is often related to acute injury or trauma, and acts as a warning system in the body.[3] Procedural pain is example of acute pain. Resolution of acute pain results from tissue healing or repair.[8]

It is imperative that health care professionals strive to have optimal pain management outcomes because acute pain that persists can transition to chronic pain, otherwise known as pain chronification.[8] Physiologic changes can occur, resulting in peripheral and central sensitization. Genetic and psychological responses also play a role in pain chronification.[8] Therefore, appropriate and timely pain management care is essential for long-term patient outcomes.

Chronic pain is currently defined as continuous or intermittent pain that continues after anticipated time for healing of tissues.[2,8,9] Chronic (persistent) pain represents long-term pain, 3 months or longer,[1] and is commonly associated with various disease processes, including psychological conditions.[8] In some cases, the causative factors are difficult to identify.[8] IASP recognizes common conditions associated with chronic pain (**Box 1**).[9]

Chronic pain can significantly affect quality of life. In the *Approaches to Pain Management: An Essential Guide for Clinical Leaders,* the Joint Commission recognizes "several negative impacts" patients can suffer from due to chronic pain (**Box 2**).[1]

Table 1 displays commonly associated subtypes of pain and the associated defining features. Cancer-related pain can be associated to each subtype of duration of pain classification.[2]

Pathophysiological

The Pathophysiological Pain classification system is based on the pathophysiological mechanism of injury to the body resulting in pain. The 2 major physiologic pathways are nociceptive and neuropathic. Nociceptive pain is a normal bodily response to injury and can result from damaged tissues, such as internal organs, muscles, and/or bone.[8,10]

Fig. 2 displays further breakdown of nociceptive pain. The 2 major categories of nociceptive pain are somatic and visceral. Somatic pain refers to injuries to the musculoskeletal system, including skin, muscles, and bone.[2] A superficial somatic injury can result from a small cut on the surface of the skin.[2] An example of deep somatic injury is a hip fracture. Visceral pain, also known as referred pain, correlates with internal organ tissues and can be felt indirectly.[1]

Pain is often associated with the inflammatory response because it aids in the healing process.[11] Persistent inflammation needs to be addressed and managed accordingly to reduce the risk of developing pathologic bodily responses. Secondary diseases and conditions associated with persistent inflammation include rheumatoid arthritis, certain cancers, and atherosclerosis.[11]

According to UpToDate, "Neuropathic pain arises from abnormal neural activity secondary to disease, injury, or dysfunction of the nervous system."[9] Neuropathic pain results from a lesion that affects the central or peripheral nervous system[8] and can be further divided into 3 subgroups: sympathetically mediated, peripheral, or central.[9] Symptoms of neuropathic pain include altered sensations, including numbness, tingling, burning, and shooting pains.[8] Examples of common conditions associated with neuropathic pain include diabetic neuropathy, human immunodeficiency virus, and phantom limb pain.[2] **Table 2** lists pain descriptor terms for neuropathic pain.[9]

Box 1
Common sources of chronic pain

- Cancer pain
- Arthritis
- Headache
- Low back pain
- Human immunodeficiency virus
- Neuropathic pain disorders

Data from International Association for the Study of Pain (IASP). Curriculum outline on pain for nursing-IASP. 2017. Available at: http://www.iasp-pain.org/Education/CurriculumDetail.aspx?ItemNumber=2052. Accessed March 9, 2017.

Box 2
Potential negative impacts of chronic pain

- Lack of sleep
- Impaired attentiveness
- Decreased mobility
- Increased weakness
- Anxiety
- Depression
- Inter-relationship issues
- Addiction to prescription pain pills
- Decreased immune function
- Work attendance issues
- Failure to hold employment
- Financial hardships

Adapted from the Joint Commission. Approaches to pain management: an essential guide for clinical leaders. 2010. Available at: http://www.jointcommissioninternational.org/assets/1/14/APM10_Sample_Pages2.pdf. Accessed March 9, 2017.

Psychological and Spiritual Aspects of Pain Classification

Recognizing the psychological impacts of pain is vital to providing holistic patient care. Physiologic changes can occur because of a patient's behavioral response to pain. According to the WHO, it is necessary to provide a holistic approach to care, which includes consideration of the individual's "sensory, physiologic, cognitive, affective, behavioral and spiritual components."[2]

The ANA recognizes several subtypes of psychological responses to painful stimulus, including fear-avoidance and catastrophizing.[8] Fear-avoidance occurs when a patient has irrational fears that activities will trigger more pain; therefore, the activities are avoided, furthering debility.[8] Catastrophizing occurs when the patient dwells on the worst possible outcomes; therefore, limits activities and reports high pain levels.

Table 1
Duration

Type	Defining Features
Acute	Short-term: <3–6 mo
Chronic	Continues after ordinary timeframe for healing of tissues
Episodic	Recurrent, can be long-term
Breakthrough	Acute, short-term; > initial pain intensity level, includes incident and end-of-dose failure
Incident	Varies, associated with movement
End of Dose	Beyond half-life; no longer effectively achieving pain goal

Adapted *from* WHO guidelines on the pharmacological treatment of persisting pain in children with medical illnesses. Geneva (Switzerland): World Health Organization; 2012. Available at: https://www.ncbi.nlm.nih.gov/books/NBK138356/. Accessed February 12, 2017; and Pain management nursing: scope and standards of practice. 2nd edition. Silver Spring (MD): American Nurses Association; 2016.

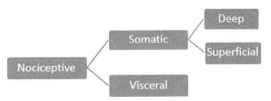

Fig. 2. Nociceptive pathway. (*Data from* WHO guidelines on the pharmacological treatment of persisting pain in children with medical illnesses. Geneva (Switzerland): World Health Organization; 2012. Available at: https://www.ncbi.nlm.nih.gov/books/NBK138356/. Accessed February 12, 2017.)

This is also correlated with debility.[8] Two common psychological disorders that are frequently associated with chronic (persistent) pain are depression and anxiety.[8] Identifying the correct classification of pain is imperative in a comprehensive pain assessment approach.[8]

Other

The classification of other category represents causes of pain syndromes that are not easily classifiable; the mechanism or pathways of the pain are not well understood. Idiopathic pain is not easily classifiable because there is no distinguishable cause for pain.[2] Cancer pain is not easily classifiable and is often associated with mixed pain. Mixed pain results from simultaneously experiencing nociceptive and neuropathic pain.[2] Additional examples of disorders that are not easily classifiable include fibromyalgia and primary headaches.[12]

PAIN CLASSIFICATION IN CLINICAL PRACTICE

To identify a timely and evidence-based plan of care before beginning treatment, utilization of the pain classification systems is necessary. The following case study of B.B. demonstrates the use of pain classifications system in clinical practice and provides a holistic view of the patient's needs, transitional states of pain, and how each classification assists with the assessment and evaluation of care. Key issues, such as barriers to and controversies in pain management, are addressed.

CASE STUDY

B.B. sustained a lifting injury to her lower back 7 months ago. She did not seek medical care until her pain was causing her to miss work days. She was eventually seen by her

Table 2	
Pathophysiological classification (neuropathic)	
Type	**Definition**
Allodynia	Pain resulting from a stimulus that does not normally elicit pain
Dysesthesia	Unpleasant abnormal sensation, whether spontaneous or evoked
Hyperalgesia	Increased response to a stimulus that normally is painful
Hypoalgesia	Diminished response to a normally painful stimulus
Hypoesthesia	Diminished sensitivity to stimulation
Paresthesia	Abnormal sensation, whether spontaneous or evoked

Data from Rosenquist EWK, Aronson MD, Crowley M. Definition and pathogenesis of chronic pain. 2017. Available at: http://www.uptodate.com/contents/definition-and-pathogenesis-of-chronic-pain. Accessed April 25, 2017.

doctor 8 weeks postinjury for throbbing, lower mid-back pain (rated 9/10 on numeric rating scale) not relieved with acetaminophen. She was given a 2-week supply of Percocet. As a consequence of missing too many work days from pain, she lost her job and health insurance. Unable to afford a follow-up visit, B.B. continued to have persistent back pain and started "borrowing" Percocet from elderly family members.

Seven months later, B.B. presented to the emergency room (ER) with sudden lower abdominal cramping (rated 10/10 on numeric rating scale) aggravated with walking, and nausea and vomiting. She cried, stating, "I have not been able to have a bowel movement for a week and when I do have a bowel movement, it is very hard, like little marbles." She complains of increased agitation and episodes of crying and feelings of anxiety over the last 6 months. Imaging and radiographs show fecal impaction. The fecal mass is broken up with digital examination and enema. B.B. is diagnosed with anxiety and constipation. She is discharged from the ER with a prescription for alprazolam and docusate sodium. Instructions are given to follow-up with primary care provider (PCP) within 2 weeks.

B.B. does not have health insurance, so is seen 2 weeks later in the community health department. A history, comprehensive pain assessment, focused examination, and identification of pain classification are completed. The family nurse practitioner's subjective, objective, assessment, and plan (SOAP) note follows.

Subjective

Patient is a 43-year-old Asian American with no history of chronic medical problems until 7 months ago. Requesting follow-up from ER 2 weeks ago. Constipation has improved. Today complains of dull, lower-back pain bilaterally (rated 6/10 on numeric rating scale) without radiation. This pain started 7 months ago after lifting greater than 40 pounds. Delayed seeing PCP for 2 months and was given 14 days Percocet 5 mg at that visit. No follow-up due to lack of insurance. Pain on most days (rated 4–6/10 on numeric rating scale), worse in morning. Denies fevers, swollen or tender joints in hands, wrists, shoulders, knees, or ankles. Denies numbness or tingling in extremities. Continues to take Percocet (10 mg). Obtains from elderly relatives. Takes 1 every 4 to 5 hours as needed on average 5 days a week with some relief. Denies history of visiting pain clinic. Complains of feeling down past few months and decreased sleep, states pain interferes with doing house chores. Has only taken alprazolam twice in past month, does not like to take due to "loopy feeling." Smokes half a pack day for 20 years. Denies alcohol or illicit drug use. Lost job recently. Recent weight gain10 pounds Spends most of time at home; denies social activities. No religion. Denies suicidal thoughts. Family history is positive for depression.

Current medications
- Oxycodone/acetaminophen, 10 mg/325 mg, 1 every 4 to 5 hours as needed for pain (not prescribed for patient; obtaining from elderly family)
- Alprazolam 0.5 mg as needed (last dose 2 weeks ago)
- Docusate sodium 100 mg, 1 by mouth twice daily.

Vitals: pain 6/10, weight 145 lb, height 64 in, blood pressure 132/84, respiration 14, temperature: 98.2°F.

Objective

Patient is dressed appropriately, talking appropriately, ambulating without problems, no apparent distress while sitting. Sad affect. Oriented times 3. Limited range of motion of lumbar spine flexion 45°, extension 15°, side-bending 20°, rotation 20°, facial grimacing with flexion of spine, no point tenderness with palpation of lower spine. Neurologically intact. No other significant physical findings.

Diagnostic tests: urinalysis normal; imaging from recent ER visit showed fecal impaction.

Screening questionnaires: SOAAP (Screener and Opioid Assessment for Patients with Pain), negative; PHQ-9 (Patient Health Questionnaire for depression), score 10.

Assessment

Chronic lower back pain (>6 month's duration); moderate depression; history constipation; tobacco dependence.

Differential diagnoses: thyroid or other metabolic disorder; anemia, substance abuse or dependence; degenerative disc disease; osteoarthritis.

Plan

Chronic lower back pain: taper Percocet (10% decrease in dose per week) and then discontinue. Start Ibuprofen 800 mg by mouth 3 times daily for 2 weeks. Discontinue alprazolam. Increase exercise. List of back strengthening or stretching exercises given to patient. Education regarding chronic pain and the benefits of using nonopioid pain-reliever versus the risks of dependence or abuse with long-term opioid use. Patient agrees to try a NSAID (nonsteroidal anti-inflammatory drug) and will report any withdrawals. Goals are to remain active, increase sleep, and decrease pain 25% by next visit.

Moderate depression: fluoxetine 20 mg by mouth daily; arrange psychological counseling.

Constipation: increase water, fiber; continue docusate sodium 100 mg twice daily. Add MiraLAX.

Tobacco use: tobacco cessation techniques discussed; patient declines.

Initial laboratory tests: CBC (complete blood count), CMP (comprehensive metabolic panel), (hemoglobin) A1C, TSH (thyroid-stimulating hormone); lumbar X-ray (radiograph).

Patient should return to clinic for re-evaluation in 2 weeks or sooner if symptoms worsen. Any thoughts of harming self or others should be reported immediately. Consider pain management specialist if pain worsens or function does not increase.

CLASSIFYING PAIN

Classifying pain is helpful in guiding the provider's assessment and in choosing the appropriate classification of analgesic for pain management. In this case study, B.B. initially started having lower back pain after her lifting injury but did not seek care until 8 weeks later. The treatment goals in cases of acute pain are early intervention, improved function, treatment of any underlying physical or emotional disorder, and decrease in the intensity of pain so to prevent changes that can occur in the nervous system, which may lead to chronic pain.[13] In 90% of patients, acute back pain will resolve within 6 weeks.[13,14] The remainder of patients will develop chronic pain.

In this case study, the goal of early intervention was not met. The patient did not initiate medical care until 8 weeks following the injury. Then, she unfortunately lost her health insurance and was unable to follow-up. B.B. succumbed to drug diversion from older family members, which led to misuse. As a result of using opioids, B.B. developed constipation, which subsequently resulted in an ER visit.

The progression of B.B.'s pain led to the classification of chronic pain, or pain lasting more than 6 months. The goals of treatment of this classification are to decrease pain and restore physical, emotional, and social function, as well as improve coping skills.[13] Many factors can contribute to chronic pain (eg, depression) and treating these underlying diseases is important in reducing pain.[15,16] A valid predictor of low back pain outcomes is the presence of emotional distress and psychosocial factors.[16] **Table 3** classifies the 3 types of pain experienced in this case study.

Chronic Pain

Currently, the United States is having a prescription opioid overdose epidemic; overdoses from opioids account for more than 90 deaths per day.[18–20] The leading cause of injury death is drug overdose death.[21] Office visits due to pain account for 20% of outpatient visits and 12% of total prescriptions written.[22] The amount of prescription opioids sold in the United States has almost quadrupled since 1999.[20]

Chronic pain is a significant medical and social issue. Pain affects everyone: patients, families, workforce, and all populations in society.[22] Importantly, pain can be more prevalent and disabling in vulnerable populations (ie, racial and ethnic minorities, those with low income or education, the elderly).[8,19] The case study presents B.B. as an Asian American and certain races (eg, Asians) have CYP2D6 allelic variants, which lead to poor metabolism of opioids and, therefore, they may not experience adequate pain relief (nonopioids are not affected by these variants).[23,24]

Physical and psychological effects from chronic pain are numerous. As in the case study, common effects include functional disability, anxiety, depression, and sleep deprivation.[22] Pain affects activities of daily living and negatively affects personal relationships.[22] Chronic pain interferes with work productivity and is the leading cause of long-term disability; more than 50 million work days are lost annually.[22] The expense to taxpayers and employers is more than $100 billion annually.[22]

Table 3
Multimodal approach to pain management

Type	PCP	ER	Health Department
Anatomic	Lower back	Lower abdominal and rectal	Generalized lower back
Etiologic	Nonmalignant pain r/t acute musculoskeletal injury	Nonmalignant pain r/t opioid use	Nonmalignant pain r/t back injury 7 mo ago
Intensity	• Numeric rating scale: 9/10 (severe) • Throbbing without radiation • Aggravated by sitting prolonged periods of time • Pain not relieved with acetaminophen	Numeric rating scale: 10/10 (severe) • Associated NV • Cramping for 10 h; dull, nagging pain for 1 wk • Aggravated by walking • Pain not relieved with Percocet	• Numeric rating score: 6/10 (moderate) • Dull without radiation • Aggravated with spinal flexion • Slight relief with Percocet
Duration	Acute (2 mo)	Acute (1 wk)	Chronic (7 mo)
Pathophysiological	Nociceptive, somatic	Nociceptive, visceral	Nociceptive, somatic
Pain Mechanism	NA	NA	Central sensitization[17]
Psychological	NA	Anxiety	Depression

Abbreviations: NA, not applicable; NV, nausea and vomiting; r/t, related to.

Prescription opioids include codeine, fentanyl, hydrocodone, hydromorphone, methadone, morphine, oxycodone, and oxymorphone.[18] Treatment of acute pain with these drugs often leads to long-term opioid use.[25] It is recommended that 3 days or less of an immediate-release opioid be prescribed for acute pain.[25] Evidence is lacking for the benefits of treating chronic pain with opioids (except for adults older than 18 years who are experiencing cancer, palliative, or end-of-life care).[20]

Chronic pain should be managed with a multimodal approach using nonopioid and nonpharmacological modalities (ie, NSAIDs, acetaminophen, remaining active, exercise, weight loss, cognitive behavioral therapy).[20,25] The use of opioids obtained through prescriptions can lead to misuse and abuse, adverse side effects (eg, constipation is most common adverse effect), drug dependency and diversion, and even fatal overdoses.[22,26] In the case study, B.B. was given 2 weeks of an opiate for acute pain and this led to constipation, diversion, and misuse.

SUMMARY

Pain classification systems are essential components for on-going assessment and evaluation of patients experiencing pain. The case study is presented to demonstrate the use of pain classification systems through a multimodal approach (see **Table 3**) and to highlight potential negative consequences and barriers in pain management. Highlighted negative consequences and barriers to care presented include socioeconomic burdens (loss of job, no insurance, lack of care), increased health care management costs (ER visit), genetic factors (Asian CYP2D6 allelic variants), psychological aspects (anxiety and depression), prescribed narcotic misuse (Percocet), opioid side effects (fecal impaction), and the addiction epidemic.

Therefore, careful attention must be given to the individual experiencing pain, with consideration of the pain classifications, negative consequences, and barriers to pain management. This will ensure a holistic approach for optimal patient care.

REFERENCES

1. Porche RA. Approaches to pain management: An essential guide for clinical leaders. The Joint Commission International. 2010. Available at: http://www.jointcommissioninternational.org/assets/1/14/APM10_Sample_Pages2.pdf. Accessed March 9, 2017.

2. WHO guidelines on the pharmacological treatment of persisting pain in children with medical illnesses. Geneva (Switzerland): World Health Organization; 2012. Available at: https://www.ncbi.nlm.nih.gov/books/NBK138356/. Accessed February 12, 2017.

3. Wurhman E, Cooney MF. Acute pain: assessment and treatment. Medscape. 2011. Available at: http://www.medscape.com/viewarticle/735034. Accessed March 9, 2017.

4. Pain. National Institutes of Health. 2016. Available at: https://nccih.nih.gov/health/pain. Accessed February 12, 2017.

5. AAPM facts and figures on pain. The American Academy of Pain Medicine. Available at: http://www.painmed.org/patientcenter/facts-on-pain/. Accessed February 12, 2017.

6. Cole BE. Pain management: classifying, understanding, and treatment pain. Hosp Physician 2002;38(6):23–30. Available at: http://www.turner-white.com/pdf/hp_jun02_pain.pdf. Accessed February 12, 2017.

7. Pain assessment scales. PainEdu improving pain through education. The National Institute of Pain Control. Available at: https://www.painedu.org/downloads/nipc/pain%20assessment%20scales.pdf. Accessed March 9, 2017.

8. Pain management nursing: scope and standards of practice. 2nd edition. Silver Spring (MD): American Nurses Association; 2016.

9. IASP curriculum outline on pain for nursing - IASP. IASP-International Association for the Study of Pain. Available at: http://www.iasp-pain.org/Education/CurriculumDetail.aspx?ItemNumber=2052. Accessed March 9, 2017.

10. Urden LD, Stacy KM, Lough ME. Critical care nursing: diagnosis and management. 6th edition. St Louis (MO): Mosby Elsevier; 2010.

11. Nordqvist C. Inflammation: causes, symptoms and treatment. Medical News Today. 2015. Available at: http://www.medicalnewstoday.com/articles/248423.php. Accessed March 9, 2017.

12. Backonja M, Dahl J, Jordan D, et al. Pain management. Classification of pain - Pain management. 2010. Available at: http://projects.hsl.wisc.edu/GME/PainManagement/session2.4.html. Accessed April 25, 2017.

13. National Pharmaceutical Council. Pain: current understanding of assessment, management, and treatments. 2001. Available at: http://www.npcnow.org/system/files/research/download/Pain-Current-Understanding-of-Assessment-Management-and-Treatments.pdf. Accessed April 23, 2017.

14. Domino FJ, Baldor RA, editors. The 5-minute clinical consult premium print online 2014. 22nd edition. Philadelphia: Wolters Kluwer Health/Lippincott Williams & Wilkins; 2014.

15. McHugh RK, Nielsen S, Weiss RD. Prescription drug abuse: from epidemiology to public policy. J Subst Abuse Treat 2015;48(1):1–7.

16. Chou R, Qaseem A, Snow V, et al. Diagnosis and treatment of low back pain: a joint clinical practice guideline from the American College of Physicians and the American Pain Society. Ann Intern Med 2007;147(7):478–91. Available at: http://annals.org/aim/article/736814/diagnosis-treatment-low-back-pain-joint-clinical-practice-guideline-from. Accessed April 25, 2017.

17. CDC. Understanding the epidemic. Centers for Disease Control and Prevention. 2016. Available at: https://www.cdc.gov/drugoverdose/epidemic/index.html. Accessed April 21, 2017.

18. McAllister M. Understanding chronic pain. Institute for Chronic Pain; 2012. Available at: http://www.instituteforchronicpain.org/understanding-chronic-pain/what-is-chronic-pain/central-sensitization. Accessed April 23, 2017.

19. US Dept. of Health & Human Services (HHS). National pain strategy. National Institutes of Health; 2016. Available at: https://iprcc.nih.gov/National_Pain_Strategy/NPS_Main.htm. Accessed April 23, 2017.

20. CDC. Opioid overdose. Centers for Disease Control and Prevention. 2017. Available at: http://www.cdc.gov/drugoverdose/prescribing/clinical-tools.html. Accessed April 23, 2017.

21. US Department of Health & Human Services. About the epidemic. HHS.gov. 2017. Available at: https://www.hhs.gov/opioids/about-the-epidemic/. Accessed April 23, 2017.

22. Rosenquist EWK, Aronson MD, Crowley M. Definition and pathogenesis of chronic pain. 2015. Available at: http://www.uptodate.com/contents/definition-and-pathogenesis-of-chronic-pain. Accessed April 25, 2017.

23. Dean L. Codeine therapy and CYP2D6 genotype. Medical genetics summaries. 2017. Available at: http://www.ncbi.nlm.nih.gov/books/NBK100662/. Accessed April 21, 2017.

24. Smith HS. Opioid metabolism. Mayo Clin Proc 2009;84(7):613–24.
25. Surgeon General of the United States. Treatment options. TurnTheTideRX. Available at: http://turnthetiderx.org/treatment/. Accessed April 23, 2017.
26. Swegle J, Logeman C. Management of common opioid-induced adverse effects. Management of common opioid-induced adverse effects - American Family Physician. 2006. Available at: http://www.aafp.org/afp/2006/1015/p1347.html. Accessed April 23, 2017.

Postoperative Visual Analog Pain Scores and Overall Anesthesia Patient Satisfaction

Tony Burch, DNAP, CRNA[a],*, Scott J. Seipel, PhD[b], Nina Coyle, BSPH[c],
Keri H. Ortega, DNAP, CRNA[d], Ozzie DeJesus, DNAP, CRNA[d]

KEYWORDS

- Patient satisfaction • Pain management • Anesthesia

KEY POINTS

- Patient satisfaction is evolving into an important measure of high-quality health care.
- Pain management is an integral part of anesthesia care and must be assessed to determine patient satisfaction; therefore, it is a measure for quality of care.
- There is no clear evidence to support a direct relationship between patient satisfaction with the anesthetic care received and pain control.
- Based on the results of this study, reported level of pain is not a consistent solo predictor for overall anesthesia patient satisfaction.
- This study shows anesthesia providers that postoperative pain is not a dominant measure in determining anesthesia patient satisfaction.

INTRODUCTION

Patient satisfaction is evolving into an important measure of high-quality health care. Anesthesia care is no exception to this quality measure. Pain management is an integral part of anesthesia care and must be assessed to determine patient satisfaction; therefore, it is a measure for quality of care. Health care has undergone tremendous legislative changes since the Patient Protection and Affordable Care Act (PPACA) of 2010. The PPACA initiated the Hospital Value-Based Purchasing Program. Program objectives are to incentivize quality rather than quantity of health care. The Hospital Consumer Assessment of Healthcare Providers and Systems

[a] 3419 Shady Forest Drive, Murfreesboro, TN 37128, USA; [b] Department of Computer Information Systems, Jones College of Business, Middle Tennessee State University, Business Aerospace Building N358, MTSU Box 45, Murfreesboro, TN 37132, USA; [c] 2614 Sunset Place, Nashville, TN 37212, USA; [d] Wolford College, 1336 Creekside Boulevard, Suite 2, Naples, FL 34108, USA
* Corresponding author.
E-mail address: tony.e.burch@gmail.com

Crit Care Nurs Clin N Am 29 (2017) 419–426
http://dx.doi.org/10.1016/j.cnc.2017.08.003
0899-5885/17/© 2017 Elsevier Inc. All rights reserved.

(HCAHPS) is a survey designed to provide a nationally standardized indicator of patients' hospital experiences. As of 2013, HCAHPS and its use as an indicator of hospital performance became mandatory according to the Centers for Medicare and Medicaid Services (CMS). A total of 1% to 2% of funds for each hospital over the next several years is being linked to how well hospitals perform on the HCAHPS.

The evaluation of quality data concerning pain and patient satisfaction has future CMS reimbursement advantages and informs anesthesia providers about the quality of care they provide. Various institutions manage pain differently. One concern regarding pain management is how patients believe their immediate postoperative pain is being managed. Another pain management issue is how patients reflect individual experiences into their overall anesthesia experience. There are several factors that contribute to patient satisfaction with their overall anesthesia care. There is a great need to determine what role postoperative pain plays in patient satisfaction related to anesthesia care satisfaction. There is a need to identify how postoperative pain scores correlate with anesthesia patient satisfaction survey results. There is limited knowledge identifying how patients correlate the anesthesia provided with immediate postoperative pain.

The anesthesia provider can use these data for multiple purposes. Financially, these data could prove valuable when requesting reimbursement from CMS or other insurance companies. These data could provide anesthesia groups or companies the ability to show stakeholders the quality of care they currently provide. This could assist with anesthesia group mergers and acquisitions throughout the health care community. Data of this nature will allow the anesthesia community to develop focused interventions that improve quality of care. These data can provide insight to improving quality of care by identifying immediate postoperative pain as a major predictor of patient satisfaction or by identifying that it is not a major predictor of anesthesia-specific patient satisfaction. The purpose of this article is to assess how postoperative visual analog scale (VAS) scores for pain compare with anesthesia patient satisfaction survey scores.

REVIEW OF LITERATURE

After reviewing the literature, there is inconsistent evidence concerning patient satisfaction and pain. Hanna and colleagues[1] (2012) performed a study that examined the relationship between patients' perceptions of pain control during hospitalization and their overall satisfaction with care. Satisfaction data were collected using the federally mandated HCAHPS survey for 4349 adult patients admitted to any surgical unit over an 18-month period. Descriptive analysis and basic bivariate analyses were conducted to account for variables on overall satisfaction.[1] Logistic regression models were used to adjust for odds ratios and statistical significance was set at $P<.01$. Statistically significant findings included that patient satisfaction was 4.86 times greater if pain was controlled. This study also concluded that patient satisfaction was 9.92 times greater if the patient considered the health care team actions to relieve pain as effective.[1]

An older study by Donovan[2] (1983), examined the attitudes of general surgical patients and the management of their postoperative pain. This study involved 200 patients from 5 different surgical units. Patients participated in a survey by the same independent interviewer. There were no statistically significant parameters set for this study. Percentages and findings were based on the patients' answers to the survey. This study found that 75% of postoperative patients reported significant pain and 86% of them conveyed they were satisfied with their pain relief.[2]

Another study by Weis and colleagues[3] (1983) examined attitudes of patients, house staff, and nurses toward postoperative analgesic care. This study included 100 patients, 97 physicians, and 142 nurses who completed a questionnaire composed of multiple-choice questions. There were no statistically significant parameters set for this study. Percentages and findings were based on the patients' answers to the survey. This study reported that 43% of patients rated their pain level as moderate to severe; 75% of those patients reported they were satisfied with their postoperative pain relief.[3]

Similarly, a more recent study by Chung and Lui[4] (2003) examined postoperative current pain intensity, most intense pain experienced, satisfaction with postoperative pain management, and the differences regarding pain and satisfaction levels. Two questionnaires were given to 294 patients who were admitted for surgery. The first questionnaire was a demographic data sheet and the second unnamed questionnaire was developed by the American Pain Society and assessed patient outcomes regarding pain. Descriptive statistics were calculated to summarize the subjects' demographic characteristics, current and worst pain intensity, and level of satisfaction with care for pain provided.[4] Mann-Whitney U tests were conducted to examine the differences in reported pain intensity based on demographic variables.[4] Analysis of variance (ANOVA) with post hoc tests were used to show the differences among clinical units regarding reported pain and satisfaction rating levels.[4] The investigators found that 85% of postoperative patients reported various levels of pain, but greater than 65% recorded their satisfaction with the pain management received.

Another study by[5] Apfelbaum and colleagues (2003) examined patients' attitudes and concerns about postoperative pain. Data was gathered via telephone questionnaires from a random sample of 250 adults that had undergone a recent surgical procedure. Percentages were calculated based on the total number of patients who answered each question. The data for this study were analyzed using descriptive statistics. Apfelbaum and colleagues[5] (2003) reported that those patients who experienced pain and received pain medications before discharge revealed they were either very satisfied or satisfied 88% of the time.

Conflicting results by other studies include findings that patients with the highest reported pain intensity score were the most dissatisfied with their pain management. Miaskowski and colleagues[6] (1994) examined patient satisfaction with pain management as a component of a total quality assurance program. This study used the patient satisfaction survey recommended by the Quality Assurance Committee of the American Pain Society. Seventy-two medical-surgical patients were questioned about their pain management. Pearson product-moment correlations were used to statistically calculate findings. This study supports that a relationship exists between pain control and patient satisfaction.

Stahmer and colleagues[7] (1998) performed a study to correlate pain intensity with pain relief and satisfaction with pain management. This study was a prospective, single-group repeated-measures design. A convenience sample of 81 patients was used and data were gathered based on VAS scores and numerical descriptor scale (NDS) scores. Agreement between the VAS and NDS scores was determined by an interclass correlation coefficient. ANOVA was used to assess differences in variables of pain intensity, initial pain score, and pain relief. To assess the relationship between pain management satisfaction and pain relief, a 1-way ANOVA was implemented. Stahmer and colleagues[7] (1998) reported that patient satisfaction is associated with the amount of pain relief achieved.

Kelly[8] (2000) assessed the relationship between pain management, patient satisfaction, and pain scores using VAS scores. This study was a prospective observational study of 54 patients in the emergency department (ED) experiencing pain. Data were gathered for this study by questioning patients and using VAS scores. Percentages were calculated based on the total number of patients who answered each question. Kelly[8] (2000) found that 70% of patients rated the management of their pain as "good" or "very good." This study concluded that patient satisfaction is not related to initial VAS score, VAS score at discharge, or changes in VAS scores from presentation to discharge. According to Kelly[8] (2000), information about the quality of analgesia provided in an ED cannot be inferred from patient satisfaction surveys.

A more recent 2013 study by Phillips and colleagues[9] examined the relationship between the level of pain control and patient satisfaction. This study involved 88 patients who received opioid analgesics. Data were obtained by using a 14-point question survey adapted from the American Pain Society. Spearman's rank correlation coefficients were calculated to determine the relationship between patients' level of pain and pain control. The bivariate correlation coefficient was determined to be $r = -0.31$ (95% CI -0.79–0.39). Phillips and colleagues[9] (2013) found there is no correlation between level of pain control and patient satisfaction.

METHODS

This project focused on correlating immediate postoperative VAS for pain scores with anesthesia patient satisfactions scores. The design is an original research study that will benefit the anesthesia community. Anesthesia providers will be able to recognize the influence postoperative pain has on patient satisfaction. With patient satisfaction being a quality measure, these data will help anesthesia providers in validating their delivery of quality care. These data could substantiate the quality of care delivered, which could delineate best-evidenced based practices for the future. This information can be further used to develop postoperative pain management algorithms or interventions until quality measures are consistent and successfully met. The problem has been identified as a need for anesthesia-specific patient satisfaction scores that positively or negatively correlate with immediate postoperative pain control.

Specific methods of this project to gather satisfaction data include patients who were surveyed using the Anesthesia Patient Satisfaction Questionnaire (APSQ). The APSQ is a 23-question tool commercially available to anesthesia practices. The APSQ was developed and administered by SurveyVitals (9g Enterprises, Inc, Springtown, TX, USA). Surveys were distributed postoperatively to all patients using a series of text messages and Interactive Voice Response telephone calls, with contact attempts terminated after survey completion or patient opt-out. Patients were asked to provide feedback to yes-or-no questions and Likert Scale (1–5) prompts. For this study, 1 month of retrospective data were pulled for analysis. Specifically, yes or no responses were gathered in response to the question, "Did you experience more pain than expected after your surgery?" and Likert scale responses were gathered for an overall rating of the anesthesia provider.

Data for VAS scores were retrospectively reviewed for the same 1-month period. Scores were obtained by the scanning of so-called bubble sheets or Data Collection Forms. Clinical staff in postanesthesia care units documented patient responses for highest recorded VAS score and VAS score at discharge. Then, the data collection forms were returned to a single administrative location for scanning into a Clinical Quality Database.

All patient, provider, and facility identifiers were removed from the data sets before reporting. A unique key for each case was used to combine patient satisfaction responses with postanesthesia care unit quality data. This study was granted an exemption by the Internal Review Board because the data available for analysis were already de-identified by the quality coordinator on receipt by the author. Once the data were compiled, the analysis phase of the project began. Statistical comparisons, analyzing relationships between postoperative VAS scores and anesthesia patient satisfaction scores were statistically analyzed and interpreted by a statistician. Interpretation included data tables to elucidate the findings.

This type of research was chosen for multiple reasons. Anesthesia providers need these data to ensure that quality patient care is being delivered.[10] With reimbursement trending toward quality of care, anesthesia providers need data to support the quality of care delivered.[10] These data may spawn other areas of specific patient satisfaction and anesthesia quality-of-care research. This project took place in a large nonprofit facility licensed for 683 acute and rehab care beds. The facility contains 2 separate main operating room areas and 2 separate ambulatory surgery centers. This project was based solely within this facility.

RESULTS
Patients

Records of 16,120 patients were evaluated. Among those who responded to the survey, 533 patients recorded valid scores on the survey instrument for both the 5-point rating scale of the quality of care and the presence of postoperative pain. Such attrition can be attributed to the need for valid responses on 2 different survey instruments. A total of 419 patients had valid VAS readings for both arrival and discharge in the data collection forms. To allow the consideration of facility effects, facilities with fewer than 8 patients in the sample were removed. This resulted in 409 total patients in the sample from 6 distinct facilities. In this final sample of 409, there were 262 patients who self-identified as female and 147 self-identified as male. The number of patients who indicated they received inpatient and outpatient treatment was 138 and 271, respectively.

Descriptive Statistics

The descriptive statistics for the results on the VAS arrival and discharge variables are shown in **Table 1**. The mean reduction in VAS from arrival to discharge was 1.78 (95% CI 1.539–2.026). The bivariate distribution of responses for the survey measurements on the quality of care and the presence of postoperative pain are shown in **Table 2**. After compressing ratings of 3 or less into a single group to address potential issues with test assumptions, a chi-square test of independence determined that there was sufficient evidence to indicate that the 2 survey responses were related ($\chi^2 = 16.507$, $df = 2$, $P = .0003$; where df is degrees of freedom).

Relationships Among Presurvey Measures

To investigate the relationship between presurvey measures, a least-squares regression was run relating the VAS at discharge to fixed (ie, gender and inpatient or outpatient) and random factors (ie, facility and VAS at arrival). The initial model showed

Table 1 Descriptive statistics		
	Mean	**Standard Deviation**
VAS on Arrival	3.31	3.307
VAS at Discharge	1.53	1.815

Table 2
Distribution of survey responses

	Postoperative Pain	
Rating of Care	Yes	No
1 (Worst)	6	3
2	4	3
3	10	2
4	14	57
5 (Best)	42	268

that the assumptions of the procedure were justifiable and a significant relationship was found (F = 42.285, df_N = 8, df_D = 400, P = .000, r^2 = .458; where F is F test). A stepwise backward protocol was used for exploration with variables not significant at the .025 level removed. The final model included the VAS at arrival (P = .000) and 1 of the facility indicator variables (P = .014). Based on this result, a partial F test was used to test the facility effect as a whole. Facilities were found to have a significant effect (F = 2.356, df_N = 5, df_D = 402, P = .040) on the VAS at discharge after controlling for VAS at arrival. No other variable was determined to have an effect on the VAS at discharge.

Relationships among survey and presurvey measures
Logistic regression was used to determine if a relationship existed between the reported postoperative pain on the survey and the presurvey variables from the patient record at discharge. No variables were considered significant contributors to the yes-or-no response from the reported postoperative pain (χ^2 = 11.036, df = 9, P = .273, Cox & Snell r^2 = .027).

Given the sparse results for quality of care, the responses for this survey were reduced to 3 ordinal categories. The transformation grouped responses of 3 or less into a single category while retaining the integrity of the original responses of 4 and 5. However, the analysis of this arrangement still proved problematic due to the assumption requirements in the application of a standard statistical procedure. To move forward in the investigation of the relationship between the quality of care and the presurvey measures, an ordinal regression was used. Because the recorded responses on the VAS measures were also sparse, these variables were also transformed into ordinal variables for the regression (**Table 3**). Transformations were not equivalent for both VAS readings because an attempt was made to equalize the number of observations in each of the new ordinal levels across VAS measures. Although there is a loss of information during the transformation into an ordinal variable, the information captured retains its primary value as a relative pain scale. Using ordinal regression, the relationship between the rating of the quality of care and the presurvey measures was evaluated. Overall model fit was significant (χ^2 = 13.881, df = 8, P = .031, Cox & Snell r^2 = .033); however, there was little evidence that a sizable part of the variability in the rating of care quality could be explained. In the full model, only the nominal variable of inpatient or outpatient status was significant (P = .005). Although the transformations necessary to create this model only resulted in the loss of information and should not have created significance where there was none, more evidence is needed to substantiate any findings of this regression.

Table 3
Transformation of visual analog scale at arrival and discharge for ordinal regression

Rating	VAS at Arrival		VAS at Discharge	
	Transformed Value	Observations	Transformed Value	Observations
0	0	172	0	194
1	0	10	0	21
2	0	18	1	72
3	0	11	1	72
4	1	18	2	31
5	1	48	2	12
6	1	53	2	1
7	2	23	2	1
8	2	36	2	1
9	2	3	2	0
10	2	17	2	4

DISCUSSION

There is no clear evidence to support a direct relationship between patient satisfaction with the anesthetic care received and pain control. The relationship between patient satisfaction and pain control presents in the literature as a multifactorial problem. According to Muller-Staub and colleagues[11] (2008) there is statistically significant correlations between worry, pain, anxiety, and patient satisfaction. Although it is publicly assumed that patients with a low VAS score would be more satisfied with their pain management when compared with patients with high VAS scores, there is not a general consensus in the literature supporting this relationship. The literature is lacking specific studies to show if a relationship exists between postoperative VAS for pain scores and overall anesthesia patient satisfaction.

Reimbursement of health care services is transitioning to reward quality rather than quantity.[10] One measure of quality is patients' experience in hospitals.[10] By determining if a relationship between postoperative VAS scores and overall patient satisfaction with anesthesia services, anesthesia providers gain knowledge to better understand the multiple variables (eg, nausea, vomiting, anxiety, privacy) involved in anesthesia patient satisfaction. Based on this study and the questionnaire, an anesthesia patient satisfaction quality indicator is generated. Analyzing and reporting these data could help ensure anesthesia patient satisfaction is consistent between facilities. Although this study concluded that reported level of pain is not a sole reliable predictor for overall anesthesia patient satisfaction, anesthesia providers can better understand the multifactorial variables associated with overall anesthesia satisfaction. Anesthesia providers could use and report these findings as a quality indicator for anesthesia services provided. Based on the results of this study, multiple quality indicators and questions should be further studied to encompass various components that affect overall anesthesia patient satisfaction.

SUMMARY

Based on the results of this study, reported level of pain is not a consistent solo predictor for overall anesthesia patient satisfaction. The results of this study suggest multiple quality indicators and questions should be further studied to encompass various components that affect overall anesthesia patient satisfaction.

To date, little research has been done to examine the direct association between postoperative VAS scores and overall anesthesia patient satisfaction. The unique component to this research is the anesthesia-specific patient satisfaction scores. The anesthesia community should assess various components that affect patient satisfaction. This study allows anesthesia providers to understand the existence of a relationship between postoperative pain and the patients' satisfaction with the overall anesthesia services received. This study shows anesthesia providers that postoperative pain is not a dominant measure in determining anesthesia patient satisfaction.

REFERENCES

1. Hanna MN, González-Fernández M, Barrett AD, et al. Does patient perception of pain control affect patient satisfaction across surgical units in a tertiary teaching hospital? Am J Med Qual 2012;27(5):411–6.
2. Donovan BD. Patient attitudes to postoperative pain relief. Anaesth Intensive Care 1983;11(2):125–9.
3. Weis OF, Sriwatanakul K, Alloza JL, et al. Attitudes of patients, housestaff, and nurses toward postoperative analgesic care. Anesth Analg 1983;62(1):70–4.
4. Chung JWY, Lui JCZ. Postoperative pain management: study of patients' level of pain and satisfaction with health care providers' responsiveness to their reports of pain. Nurs Health Sci 2003;5(1):13–21.
5. Apfelbaum JL, Chen C, Mehta SS, et al. Postoperative pain experience: results from a National survey suggest postoperative pain continues to be undermanaged. Anesth Analg 2003;97(2):534–40.
6. Miaskowski C, Nichols R, Brody R, et al. Assessment of patient satisfaction utilizing the American Pain Society's quality assurance standards on acute and cancer-related pain. J Pain Symptom Manage 1994;9(1):5–11.
7. Stahmer SA, Shofer FS, Marino A, et al. Do quantitative changes in pain intensity correlate with pain relief and satisfaction? Acad Emerg Med 1998;5(9):851–7.
8. Kelly A-M. Patient satisfaction with pain management does not correlate with initial or discharge VAS pain score, verbal pain rating at discharge, or change in VAS score in the emergency department. J Emerg Med 2000;19(2):113–6.
9. Phillips S, Gift M, Gelot S, et al. Assessing the relationship between the level of pain control and patient satisfaction. J Pain Res 2013;6:683–9.
10. Woodbury A, Williams K, Gulur P. Patients and their pain experience in the hospital: the HCAHPS imperative with payments at risk in value-based purchasing environment. ASA Newsletter 2014;78(3):28–9.
11. Muller-Staub M, Meer R, Briner G, et al. Measuring patient satisfaction in an emergency unit of a Swiss university hospital: occurrence of anxiety, insecurity, worry, pain, dyspnea, nausea, thirst and hunger, and their correlation with patient satisfaction (part 2). Pflege 2008;21:180–8.

Pharmacologic Interventions for Pain Management

Francisca Cisneros Farrar, EdD, MSN, RN*, Danielle White, MSN, RN,
Linda Darnell, MSN, RN

KEYWORDS

- Acute pain • Pain management guidelines • Pain assessment tools
- Intravenous opioid analgesics • Nonopioid analgesics • Sedative analgesics
- Benzodiazepines • Case reports

KEY POINTS

- Acute pain is a global source of distress, especially in vulnerable and compromised critically ill patients.
- Pain management requires a holistic approach that is patient centered and includes the interprofessional team.
- Nurses must acquire self-efficacy in performing a comprehensive pain assessment in verbal and nonverbal patients for evaluation of their subjective and objective pain.
- The nurse must use clinical reasoning and critical thinking skills in the administration of pain medications in a critically ill patient to prevent serious side effects and adverse reactions.
- The nurse has an ethical and legal responsibility to provide safe, quality, and accountable pain management.

INTRODUCTION

Acute pain is a universal pervasive source of distress in critically ill patients that can be treated by pharmacologic therapy, such as opioid sedative analgesic medications.[1] Most patients in the critical care setting experience pain owing to underlying illness, surgery, injury, or care interventions. Pain management for this vulnerable and compromised population requires compassion and evidence-based best practices. Pain management requires a holistic approach incorporating patient-centered care

Disclosures: There are no disclosures or conflict of interest for any relationship with a commercial company that has a direct financial interest in subject matter or materials discussed in article or with a company making a competing product.
Austin Peay State University, School of Nursing, PO Box 4658, Clarksville, TN 37043, USA
* Corresponding author.
E-mail address: farrarf@apsu.edu

to include physical, psychological, and cultural perspectives into a collaborative treatment plan.[1,2] The critical care nurse must acquire self-efficiency in conducting a comprehensive assessment for a verbal and sedated patient using evidence-based assessment tools, develop clinical reasoning skills for administering pain medications, and embrace ethical principles that serve as the foundation for their role in advocating for quality, safe, and accountable pain management for this vulnerable population.[1] This article presents a clinical toolkit for pain management that includes an ethical framework, professional guidelines, evidence-based pain assessment tools, pharmacologic medication therapy, and focused monitoring of side effects and adverse reactions. The focused population is critically ill hospitalized patients. Case reports demonstrate the application of critical thinking and clinical reasoning skills needed for pain management.

PAIN MANAGEMENT GUIDELINES

The Surgeon General's 2016 *Report on Alcohol, Drugs, and Health* points out that the United States has a serious substance misuse problem and a national opioid crisis.[3] According to the report:

- In 2015, 27.1 million people in were users of illicit drugs or misused prescription drugs.
- In 2014, 47,055 drug overdoses were reported.
- In 2014, 28,647 people died from some type of opioid overdose.
- Substance misuse costs more than $400 billion annually owing to health issues, lost productivity owing to disability, and cost of crime.
- In 2007, costs associated with the use of nonprescription medications and illegal drugs were more than $193 billion dollars
- Opioid misuse is a national public health crisis and related to overprescribing of opioid pain relievers.[3]
- A Prescription Drug Monitory Program emerged as a tool to reduce prescription drug abuse and diversion. The electronic data are used for enforcement, abuse prevention, education, and research. Currently, 49 states have legislation for the use of a Prescription Drug Monitory Program with 16 states monitoring schedules II through IV and 35 states monitoring II through V. The focus is drugs containing narcotics and tranquilizers.[3,4]

Fears of drug addiction, myths regarding opioid pain management, and social media releases about the opioid crisis distorts attitudes about pain management. It is important that the pain management nurse and the collaborative team have evidence-based education about standards of practice, their scope of practice, legal rights of patients to be treated for their pain, and perform value clarification to embrace an ethical framework to guide their pain management plan of care.

Ethical Guidelines

In 2016, The American Nurses Association (ANA) and American Society for Pain Management Nursing partnered to publish a second edition for standards of practice guidelines for pain management. These prestigious nursing organizations view the *ANA Code of Ethics for Nurses with Interpretive Statements* as the guiding ethical framework for pain management nurses.[1] Moral and ethical principles are integrated into their ethical pain management guidelines. It is important that the nurse clarify their own values and beliefs about pain management through value clarification to empower an unbiased attitude toward the care of their critically ill patients. The nurse needs to understand that what is right for him or her may not always be right for others, including patients and their families.[5]

The *ANA Code of Ethics for Nurses with Interpretive Statements* and ethical principles provide an ethical framework for pain management decision making. These 2 ethical frameworks clarify the ethical nurse practice role and the nurse's scope of practice in pain management as shown in **Table 1**.

Joint Commission on Accreditation and Healthcare Organizations Guidelines

In 2001 the Joint Commission on Accreditation of Healthcare Organizations (JCAHO and now known as the Joint Commission) responded to a national problem of undertreatment of pain by establishing standards for pain assessment and treatment for organizations involved in providing direct provision care.[2,5,6] The Rights and Ethics Standard requires health care organizations to develop policies and procedures regarding the right of patients for involvement in all aspects of their care. The Rights and Ethics Standard was incorporated into these pain management standards.[3] The following are the original standards.

- The health care organization addresses care at the end of life.
- Patients have the right to appropriate assessment and management of pain.
- Pain is assessed in all patients.
- Policies and procedures support safe medication prescription or ordering.
- The patient is monitored during the postprocedure period.
- The discharge process provides for continuing care based on the patient's assessed needs at the time of discharge.
- The organization collects data to monitor its performance.[7]

In response to pain being assessed in all patients, the American Pain Society announced pain was the fifth vital sign.[2] Some organizations such as the Veterans Administration endorsed pain as a vital sign, with pain being assesses with vital signs and recorded.[8] In 2002, the Institute for Safe Medication Practices released a report that the quest to relieve pain had compromised safety. Unintended consequences surfaced with the Joint Commission's pain management standards now that resulted in a change in the pain management standard.[9] The requirement for pain to be assessed in all patients was changed to pain is assessed and managed in patients.[6,7]

Currently with the prescription opioid epidemic, the Joint Commission's pain management standards have been targeted as a causative factor for the increased use of opioids in treating critically ill patients and discharge prescriptions for opioids for pain management.[6] On April 18, 2016, Dr David Baker, executive president for health care quality evaluation, released a statement in response to the Joint Commission's pain standards being blamed for the opioid prescription crisis.[6] In his address, the following common misconceptions leading to this blame of the Joint Commission were discussed.

- Endorses pain as a vital sign.
    Response: Do not endorse pain as a vital sign and not part of pain standards.
- Requires pain assessment for all patients.
    Response: This requirement was eliminated in 2009.
- Requires that all pain be treated until the pain score reaches zero.
    Response: Goal is for an individualized patient-centered approach that does not require zero pain.

Table 1
Nurse's scope of practice in pain management

Provision	Ethical Nurse Practice Role	Ethical Principles
1. The nurse practices with compassion and respect for the inherent dignity, work, and unique attributes of every person.	Advocacy, education, supportive approach, honor patient's right to self-determination, autonomy, and dignity, population centered care, and set aside prejudices and biases.	Autonomy Justice Beneficence Veracity
2. The nurse's primary commitment is to the patient, whether an individual, family, group, community, or population.	Kindness, respect, ensure patient acceptance, conflict resolution, interprofessional collaboration, ensure patient's autonomy and patient and public safety, maintain legal boundaries	Autonomy Fidelity Justice Nonmaleficience
3. The nurse promotes, advocates for, and protects the rights, health, and safety of the patient.	Privacy and confidentiality, trust, avoid excessive disclosure, risk evaluation, mitigation.	Autonomy Fidelity Justice
4. The nurse has authority, accountability, and responsibility for nursing practice; makes decisions; and takes action consistent with the obligation to promote health and to provide optimal care.	Interprofessional team leader, professional judgment, consultation, compliance with state nursing act, organizational policies, legal statues, rules, regulations, nursing standard of practice.	Autonomy Beneficence Nonmaleficience Fidelity Justice Veracity
5. The nurse owes the same duty to self as others, including the responsibility to promote health and safety, preserve wholeness of character and integrity, maintain competence, and continue personal and professional growth.	Duty care self, model health maintenance owing to risk moral distress, competence, lifelong learning.	Beneficence Nonmaleficience Veracity
6. The nurse through individual and collective effort, establishes, maintains, and improves the ethical environment of the work setting and conditions of employment that are conductive to safe, quality health care.	Moral agents, advocate, safety, evidence-based plan of care.	Autonomy Beneficence Nonmaleficience Fidelity Justice Veracity
7. The nurse, in all roles and settings, advances the profession through research and scholarly inquiry, professional standards development, and the generation of both nursing and health policy.	Research, scholarly inquiry, dissemination of knowledge and application of evidence-based guidelines, leader, mentor.	Beneficence Nonmaleficience Fidelity Justice Veracity
8. The nurse collaborates with other health professionals and the public to protect human rights, promote health diplomacy, and reduce health disparities.	Ethical obligation to advocate for equal access and prevent incongruences with disparities.	Beneficence Nonmaleficience Veracity
9. The profession of nursing, collectively through its professional organizations, must	Emulate professional nursing values, maintain integrity of profession, integrate principles of	Beneficence Nonmaleficience Justice

(continued on next page)

Table 1 (*continued*)		
Provision	**Ethical Nurse Practice Role**	**Ethical Principles**
articulate nurse values, maintain the integrity of the profession, and integrate principles of social justice into nursing and health policy.	social justice in nursing and health care policy.	Veracity

Data from American Nurses Association and American Society for Pain Management Nursing (2016). Pain management nursing: scope and standards of practice, 2nd edition. Silver Spring (MD); and Doody Q, Noonan M. Nursing research ethics, guidance and application in practice. Br J Nurs 2016;25(14):803–7.

- Standards push doctors to prescribe opioids.
  - Response: Treatment strategies for pain may include pharmacologic and nonpharmacologic approaches.
- Pain standards caused a sharp increase in opioid prescriptions.
  - Response: Claim is contradicted by data from the National Institute on Drug Abuse.[6,7]

Current standards

The Joint Commission's current standards required accredited programs to establish policies regarding pain assessment, treatment, and education. The standards do not require the use of drugs or specify which drug is prescribed. The 2017 pain management standards are currently being developed in response to the opioid crisis and criticism that Joint Commission pain management standards are a causative factor.[8,10] As a pain management nurse, it is important that you are educated about your facility's pain management policy and unit-specific policies. Many facilities have intravenous opioids and titration policies that can be downloaded as a resource. Nurses have a legal and ethical responsibility to be competent about policies and efficacy in clinical reasoning and critical thinking in assessing and evaluating patient responses to pain. Currently Joint Commission requires the following pain management guidelines.

- Conduct a comprehensive pain assessment incorporating the scope of care, patient's condition, treatment, and services needed.
- Assess pain that reflects the patient's ability to understand, condition, and age.
- Use assessment criteria to reassess and respond to the patient's pain.
- Treat the pain using a patient-centered approach and current presentation.
- Treat or refer the patient for pain treatment using pharmacologic and/or nonpharmacologic approaches.
- Pain management should include using clinical judgment about the risks and benefits with the pain management plan.
- Assess for the potential risk of dependency, addiction, and abuse.[6–8]

Medicare Guidelines

Current health care delivery models are value-based performance models. Medicare administrators responded to this financial incentive model with the establishment of never events, core measurements, and quality indicators. Hospitals receive ratings and star recognition based on meeting these performance outcome measurements. If outcomes are not met, financial constraints can be imposed, impacting financial reimbursement of patient care for hospital care. An important quality indicator that emerged is patient satisfaction. When a Medicare patient is discharged from inpatient care, a random sample of adult patients receives a patient satisfaction survey called the Hospital Consumer Assessment of Healthcare Providers and Systems (HCAHPS).[11] In April 2015, the Centers for Medicare and Medicaid Services added HCAHPS Star Ratings to the Hospital Compare website, www.medicare.gov/hospitalcompare.[11] Financial incentives are linked to this patient survey by the Centers for Medicare and Medicaid Services. Therefore, great emphasis is placed on receiving high scores on HCAHPS scores. Fifty-eight physicians who are members of the Physicians for Responsible Opioid Prescribing (PROP) signed a petition that was sent to the Centers for Medicare and Medicaid Services requesting changes to the HCAHPS Survey.[12] The petition from the physicians expressed concern that the 3 pain questions in the 32 item tool had created the unintended consequence of encouraging aggressive opioid use in hospitalized patients to treat pain and aggressive opioid prescriptions upon discharge.[12] The PROP argued that the pressure to obtain high HCAHPS scores contributed to the prescription opioid crisis, causing an unintended consequence of opioid addiction and overdose deaths.[12] The PROP wanted the following pain questions related to experiences in the hospital that range from never, sometimes, usually, and always removed.[12]

- *Question 12.* During this hospital stay, did you need medicine for pain?
- *Question 13.* During this hospital stay, how often was your pain well-controlled?
- *Question 14.* During this hospital stay, how often did the hospital staff do everything they could to help you with your pain?[13]

The PROP argued that the questions were an unrealistic expectation and nonpharmacologic methods were also available. The physicians requested a proposal for removing the 3 questions. On August 24, 2016, Sean Cavanaugh, Director for the Center of Medicare, responded in a letter to the petition supporting the PROP concerns. He reported that starting in 2018 the HCAHPS pain management dimension questions would be removed to eliminate confusion and the overprescribing of opioid medications.[14]

National Pain Management Guidelines

In 2016, the American Association and the American Society for Pain Management published a second edition, revising pain management guidelines to incorporate current issues with pain management. In addition to the guidelines from these 2 national associations, the nurse must be competent on their state board of nursing scope of practice, state law that provides rules and regulations, and their clinical practice facility's pain management policies. The following highlight significant guideline competencies for the frontline nurse at the bedside from these national pain management guidelines.[1]

- Standard 1. Assessment.
  1. Collect pertinent data and information related to patient's health, pain, or situation.
  2. Use the biopsychosocial spiritual model to collect comprehensive assessment data.

3. Involve the patient, family, significant other, and interprofessional team.
4. Use holistic, culturally sensitive, and comprehensive data collection method.
5. Include the patient's values, preferences, and expressed and unexpressed needs.
6. Recognize one's values, beliefs, and attitudes that can the impact the personal experience with pain.
7. Recognize the patient as the authority of his or her own pain by honoring patient-centered preferences.
8. Identify language barriers for effective communication.

Use valid and reliable assessment tools.[1]

- Standard 2. Diagnosis.
   1. Identify actual or potential risks.
   2. Prioritize pain-related and other diagnoses, problems, or issues.

Use appropriate pain assessment and standardized classification systems.[1]

- Standard 3. Outcome Identification.
   1. Incorporate a collaborative approach to identification of outcomes.
   2. Develop culturally sensitive expected pain-related outcomes.
   3. Generate a time frame for outcomes.
   4. Modify outcomes based on patient's pain level and situation.[1]
- Standard 4. Planning.
   1. Develop an individualized, holistic, evidence-based pain management plan in partnership with the patient, family, and interprofessional team.
   2. Advocate for a plan that minimizes unwarranted, unwanted, and suffering prevention treatment plan.
   3. Incorporate current law, rules and regulations, and standards in the plan.
   4. Consider the cost and economic implications of the plan.
   5. Modify and plan ongoing treatment based on patient's response to plan.[1]
- Standard 5. Implementation.
   1. Implement a plan appropriate to the assessment diagnosis.
   2. Interventions include integrative methods including pharmacologic and Vnon-pharmacologic interventions.
   3. Demonstrate caring, nonjudgmental behavior to develop therapies.
   4. Provide patient-centered, culturally congruent, and holistic care.[1]
- Standard 6. Evaluation.
   1. Conduct a holistic, systematic, ongoing, collaborative, and criterion-based evaluation of outcomes.
   2. Disseminate with the patient and other stakeholders in accordance with facility, state, and federal regulations.[1]
- Standard 7. Ethics.
   1. Integrate the Code of Ethics for Nurses with Interpretative Statements to guide the pain management plan.
   2. Provide care without prejudice and with compassion and respect.[1]
- Standard 8. Culturally Congruent Practice.
   1. Respect patient decisions based on cultural diversity, age, family influence, and acculturation stage.[1]
- Standard 9. Communication.
   1. Use language translation resources if language barrier present.
   2. Identify when alternative communication strategies are needed.[1]

- Standard 10. Collaboration.
  1. Collaborate with patients and other key stakeholders in developing and modifying a treatment plan.
  2. Communicate nurse's role and responsibility in collaborative team.[1]
- Standard 11. Leadership.
  1. Provide leadership in pain management plan.
  2. Accountable for delegated nursing care.[1]
- Standard 12. Education.
  1. Participate in ongoing pain management education to maintain competency.[1]
- Standard 13. Evidence-Based Practice and Research.
  1. Integrate evidence-based practice and research in plan of care.[1]
- Standard 14. Quality of Practice.
  1. Ensure patient-centered plan is timely, safe, effective, efficient, and equitable.[1]
- Standard 15. Professional Practice Evaluation.
  1. Evaluate plan to ensure pain management plan meets all regulatory requirements.[1]
- Standard 16. Resource Utilization.
  1. Use organizational and community resources to plan, provide, and sustain an interprofessional pain management plan.[1]
- Standard 17. Environmental Health.
  1. Use products and treatments to reduce environmental threats and promote safe practice environments.[1]

ASSESSMENT TOOLS

Underestimation and undertreatment of pain is a common problem in the critically ill patient especially in patients who cannot communicate.[15] In 2012, Rose and colleagues[16] surveyed 3753 intensive care unit nurses about their pain assessment and management practices with 842 nurses responding to the survey. In the study, 267 nurses (33%) used pain assessment tools for patients unable to communicate and 712 nurses (89%) used pain assessment tools for patients able to self-report.[16] The study concluded that a substantial proportion of the critical care nurses were unaware of published guidelines by professional societies. The researchers pointed out that pain assessment and management are core competencies of intensive care nurses. They recommended the need for education to improve compliance.[16]

It is extremely important that nurses caring for critically ill patients be competent about reliable and valid pain assessment tools. Nurses need orientation to unit-specific policies and measurement tools adopted by their facility. Common critically ill pain assessments are divided into self-report tools and observation tools.

Patients Who Can Communicate

Self-reported pain should be used if possible, because the patient is the best judge of the intensity and relief of pain. A comprehensive self-reported pain assessment includes pain history, location, intensity, quality, duration, aggravating factors, impact on functional ability, rating of pain intensity, patient's personal goal for pain relief, and methods of pain management that have been helpful and/or unhelpful in the past. A common self-report tool for critically ill patients is the visual analog scale, where the patient reports a discrete number on the line between 0 and 10.[15] The patient is asked to rate how the pain feels with 0 being none, 5 moderate, and 10 unbearable. The patient can also mark on the pain rating line to communicate their level of pain.[15]

Patients Who Cannot Communicate

Pain assessment in critically ill patients is challenging because of patients being compromised by altered level of consciousness and sedation.[17] If the patient is unable to provide a self-report, priority should be given to:

- Presence of pathologic conditions or procedures that usually cause pain;
- Behaviors indicating pain, such as grimacing and agitation;
- Reports of pain from parent, family, or significant other; and
- Physiologic measures such as vital signs such as tachycardia, hypertension, tachypnea, and diaphoresis.

The Behavioral Pain Scale and the Critical Care Observation Tool (CPOT) are 2 common, validated tools developed for nonverbal critically ill patients.[15] Nurses need to know both physiologic and behavioral cues of pain for efficacy in using these observation tools.[18] The PBS and CPOT both assess pain-related behaviors and physiologic indicators.[15] The Behavioral Pain Scale asks observation questions about facial expression, upper limb movements, and compliance with mechanical ventilation.[15] The CPOT is more extensive, asking observation questions about the facial expression, body movements, muscle tension evaluated by passive flexion and extension of upper extremities, compliance with the ventilator in intubated patients, and vocalization in extubated patients.[15]

A 2006 study by Chanques and colleagues[19], evaluating the impact of systematic evaluation of pain and agitation in the intensive care unit, concluded that the use of the Behavioral Pain Scale and the Richmond Agitation Sedation Scale was associated with a decrease in the incidence of pain and agitation during mechanical ventilation. Another study in 2014 by Rijkenberg and colleagues[20] compared the Behavioral Pain Scale and the CPOT in uncommunicative and sedated patients in the intensive care unit. The study concluded that the Behavioral Pain Scale and CPOT tools were both reliable and valid observation tools.[20] Arbour and Gelinas[21] (2011) recommend revising pain management protocols with the implementation of observation tools and establish cutoff scores with the CPOT tool.

CASE REPORT ON PAIN ASSESSMENT GUIDELINES AND TOOLS

RD is a 68-year-old man who was transferred to the recovery room after bilateral total knee surgery. Handoff report reveals the patient was involved in a motor vehicle accident involving a crushing injury to both knees. A postoperative pain assessment was conducted by the nurse post report. Vital signs were heart rate, 92; respiratory rate, 18; oral temperature, 98.0°F; and blood pressure, 118/70 mm Hg. The patient is drowsy but able to awaken to self-report he has a pain level of 8 of 10 and nausea. The nurse notices he is also grimacing and his heart rate is elevated, indicating a physiologic response to pain. His postoperative orders are morphine 4 to 8 mg intravenous for pain and ondansetron (Zofran) 2 mg intravenous for nausea. She identifies that the patient's age of 68 falls in the special population of elderly patients requiring a reduced morphine dose. The nurse administers morphine 4 mg intravenous and ondansetron 2 mg intravenous. Thirty minutes later, the nurse awakes RD and he is more alert with a self-report pain level of 2 of 10 and no nausea. The nurse followed pain management guidelines and was successful in managing RD's pain and nausea. Clinical reasoning was used in administering the correct medication for this vulnerable and compromised elderly patient in pain.

GENERAL CONSIDERATIONS WITH PHARMACOLOGIC INTERVENTIONS
Patient-Centered Partnership

Pain management requires a collaborative team approach that includes the patient, family, and/or significant other. A patient-centered partnership needs by be developed with patients and their support group by engaging them in the process and reinforcing the commitment to helping the patient be comfortable. Nurses rely on a self-report of pain, side effects, and adverse reactions from this shared partnership. Patient satisfaction with pain control is also associated with this caregiver patient relationship, relief of fears and anxieties, and patient involvement. **Box 1** provides tips for patient-centered care and a shared relationship.

Special Population Considerations

No 2 patients are identical; however, there are some patients that require special assessment considerations.

Prior experience with opioids

A patient with a previous or current experience with opioids will require an individualized plan for pain control owing to potential tolerance to the prescribed dose. Therefore, a higher dose of pharmacologic intervention may be needed. The regime should have an emphasis on a multimodal approach with nonopioid analgesics in combination with the opioid. The patient needs to be closely monitored for withdrawal symptoms and pain response to the treatment plan.[22,23]

Morbid obesity

Patients with morbid obesity are prone to obstructive sleep apnea and are at increased risk of respiratory depression when opioids and sedatives are administered. Pharmacologic interventions will need to be adjusted to body size, therefore requiring a higher dose. The patient needs to be closely monitored for the respiratory depression and the effects of the analgesia.[22]

Box 1
Tips for partnering with patients

1. Communicate the plan of care to include when and how to ask for medicine.

2. Tell the patient the name of the drug and the dose.

3. Explain the rationale for frequent assessment and monitoring process and the need to awaken the patient.

4. Engage the family to report negative side effects.

5. Use words that convey care and understanding.

6. Alleviate anxiety through explanations and reassurance.

7. Use nonpharmacologic measures to augment pain relief (eg, positioning, cold and heat, music, temperature control).

Data from Drew D, Gordan D, Morgan B, et al. The use of as-needed range orders for opioid analgesics in the management of pain: a consensus statement of the American society of pain management nurses and the American pain society pain management nursing. 2014. Available at: http://www.aspmn.org/documents/RangeOrderPublished2014.pdf. Accessed April 26, 2017; and Hayes K, Gordon DB. Delivering quality pain management: the challenge for nurses. AORN J 2015;101:328–34. Available at: https://www.aorn.org/websitedata/cearticle/pdf_file/CEA15508-0001.pdf. Accessed April 15, 2017.

Box 2
Side effects of opioids
Central Nervous system depressant effects
Respiratory drive depression
Hallucinations
Central and peripheral vasodilation
Histamine release
Nausea and vomiting
Hypotension
Delirium
Ileus
Urinary retention
Pruritus
Increased intracranial pressure
Data from Pandharipande P, Parsons P, Finlay G, editors. Pain control in the critically ill adult patient. Available at: www.uptodate.com. Accessed April 26, 2017.

Geriatric patients

The cognitive ability of the geriatric patient should be addressed related to pain assessment. Tools appropriate to the cognitive ability should be used in conjunction with extensive evaluation and questioning related to unreported and unrelieved pain. A geriatric patient often has differing attitudes related to pain and often suffer chronic pain from arthritis and other conditions thus making him or her less willing to report pain. Physiology in a geriatric patient alters the ways that drugs are distributed, metabolized, and excreted. Reduced doses based on age and medical health need to be considered in providing safe and effective pain medications.[22]

Side Effect Considerations

General considerations need to be considered and managed for side effects of opioids as summarized in **Box 2**. General considerations also need to be considered with focus monitoring for tolerance to high daily doses, withdrawal if on high-dose infusion for more than 1 week with the need to wean off, and a patient developing opioid-induced hyperalgesia in which the patient becomes more sensitive to painful stimuli.[15]

COMMON INTRAVENOUS SEDATIVE ANALGESICS

Intravenous opioids are the first line treatment for nonneuropathic pain with efficacy primarily owing to the mu-opioid receptor.[15] Risks, benefits, side effects, and adverse effects must be considered before selection of the specific opioid. Common intravenous sedative opioid analgesics used in pain management of acute pain in critically ill patients include morphine sulfate, fentanyl, and hydromorphone. **Boxes 3–5** overview the opioid, mechanism of action, uses, safety issues, and focused monitoring of the opioid sedative analgesic.

Box 3
Morphine Sulfate

A sedative-analgesic central nervous system opioid agent.

Mechanism of Action

Morphine sulfate binds to opioid receptors in the central nervous system promoting analgesia and respiratory depression. Binding to opioid receptors inhibits ascending pain pathways and alters the perception of and response to pain. This central nervous system response decreases brain stem respiratory centers response to carbon dioxide tension and electrical stimulation.

Uses

Common opioid used in critically ill patients for pain management as an intravenous as-needed order, patient-controlled analgesia pump, continuous infusion, epidural, and intrathecal. Morphine sulfate is used for as-needed order, patient-controlled analgesia pumps, and with continuous infusions. Astramorph/PF and Duramorph are used for epidural lumbar region infusion, and Astramorph/PF, Duramorph, and Infumorph are used with intrathecal lumbar region infusions.

Safety Issues

Black box warning for

- Serious life-threatening or fatal respiratory depression may occur.
- A single-dose of Duramorph neuraxial administration may cause acute or delayed respiratory depression for up to 24 hours.
- Misuse or erroneous substitution of Infumorph for Duramorph may result in overdose, seizures, respiratory depression, or possibly death.
- Concomitant use warning for opioids with benzodiazepines or other CNS depressants may result in profound sedation, respiratory depression, coma, and death.

Concomitant warning of opioids with serotonergic drugs may cause potential life-threatening serotonin syndrome.

Severe hypotension including orthostatic hypotension and syncope

Central nervous system depression including impaired mental and physical abilities

Focused Monitoring

Monitor for

- Central nervous system depression.
- Hypotension.
- Respiratory depression.
- Adequate analgesia is indicative of clinical efficacy.
- Toxicity; naloxone is the antidote.

Data from Refs.[15,24–27]

Box 4
Fentanyl

Fentanyl is a synthetic derivative of morphine and a sedative-analgesic central nervous system opioid agent.

It is also classified as an antilidopiperidine opioid and general anesthetic.

Mechanism of Action

Fentanyl is a pure opioid agonist of high analgesic sedative potency with immediate onset owing to its lipid solubility allowing faster penetration of the blood–brain barrier. Fentanyl compared with morphine is 80 to 100 times more potent. This opioid analgesic has less hypotension and lack of histamine release.

Uses

Fentanyl is used primarily as a continuous intravenous solution in critically ill patient. It is used in surgery for premedication, as an adjunct to general and regional anesthesia, and for postoperative pain management. Fentanyl intravenously can be administered intermittently, continuously, as patient-controlled analgesia, epidurally, and intrathecally. In the critical care setting, it is used for mechanically ventilated patients.

Safety Issues

Black box warning

- Respiratory depression during initiation and dose increase with risk of respiratory arrest.
- Concomitant use with CYP3A4 may increase effects causing potential fatal respiratory depression. If CYP3A4 discontinued can result in increased fentanyl concentrations.
- Concomitant use with warning for opioids with benzodiazepines or other central nervous system depressants may result in profound sedation, respiratory depression, coma, and death.

Medication safety issues

- Fentanyl can be confused with alfentanil and sufentanil.
- Fentanyl is among a list of drug classes by the Institute for Safe Medication Practices as a high-risk drug causing significant patient harm in a medication error.

Use with caution in head trauma patients owing to exaggerated elevation of intracranial pressure may occur.

May aggravate seizures in patients with convulsive disorders

Focused Monitoring

- Central nervous system depression.
- Hypotension/syncope.
- Respiratory depression.
- Opioid agonist toxicity; naloxone is the antidote.

Data from Refs.[15,25,27–29]

Box 5
Hydromorphone

A semisynthetic morphine derivative and sedative-analgesic central nervous system opioid agent.

Analgesic alternative option to fentanyl or morphine.

Intravenous brand name is Dilaudid.

Mechanism of Action

Binds to opioid receptors in the central nervous inhibiting ascending pain pathways, altering the perception of and response to pain, causing cough suppression, and generalized central nervous system depression. Compared with morphine, hydromorphone is 5 to 10 times more potent and is available in highly concentrated preparations. Therefore, hydromorphone is the first choice in fluid-restricted patients. Hydromorphone has a short half-life and a rapid onset within 30 minutes.

Uses

Used primarily in intravenous for treatment of moderate to severe pain in critically ill patients. Intravenous hydromorphine can be administered intermittently, continuously, as patient-controlled analgesia, and epidurally. An intermittent intravenous solution is available in a solution prefilled syringe and a solution reconstituted injection.

Safety Issues

Black box warning

- Risk of overdose or death with medication error with this high-potency sedative analgesic opioid.
- Life-threatening respiratory depression potential with start of hydromorphine and increase in dose.
- Concomitant use with warning for opioids with benzodiazepines or other central nervous system depressants may result in profound sedation, respiratory depression, coma, and death.

Safety alerts

- Parenteral alert: vial stopper may contain latex.
- Intravenous push must be given slowly over a minimum of 2 to 3 minutes.
- Hydromorphone may be confused with morphine.
- Dilaudid may be confused with Demerol and Dilantin.
- Hydromorphone is among a list of drug classes by the Institute for Safe Medication Practices as a high-risk drug, causing significant patient harm in a medication error.
- Potentially neurotoxic owing accumulation in renal or hepatic dysfunction.

Focused Monitoring

- Central nervous system depression.
- Hypotension.
- Phenanthrene hypersensitivity.
- Adequate analgesia is indicative of clinical efficacy.
- Toxicity; naloxone is the antidote.

Data from Refs.[15,25,27,30,31]

CASE REPORT REGARDING OPIOID EDUCATION

JC, a 70-year-old Hispanic man who does not speak English, fell at home and sustained an introchanteric fracture of the left hip. He has a history of hypertension, osteoporosis, osteoarthritis to both hips, and type 2 diabetes. There was no loss of consciousness during the fall. JC was admitted to the hospital for a left hemiarthroplasty surgery. After surgery, he is transferred to a surgical unit with a morphine patient-controlled anesthesia pump. His daughter, who speaks English, is with him. The nurse conducts a pain assessment with the daughter reporting his pain at 3 of 10. Education is given to JC and the daughter about the patient-controlled anesthesia pump for pain management. The daughter decides to leave for the day. The nurse returns in an hour to assess the patient. JC is unable to communicate with the nurse and is agitated. The nurse calls for an interpreter and discovers JC did not understand he could push the button for more morphine to relieve his pain. His current pain level is 7 of 10. Education is provided with the patient using the interpreter to translate the information into Spanish. JC accurately performed a return demonstration, pushing the button for extra morphine. The nurse recognized the need for an interpreter with the language barrier and that additional education with return demonstration was needed for JC to learn how to self-administer small doses of morphine with pushing the button. JC did have the manual dexterity to push the button with the observed return demonstration. It is important for nurses to assess health literacy and language barriers with the use of patient-controlled anesthesia pumps and education about opioid pain management.

COMMON ORAL OPIOIDS

Enteral opioids are effective alternatives for moderate to severe pain to allow discontinuation of intravenous opioids. Two common oral opioids used in treatment of critically ill patients are oxycodone and methadone. **Boxes 6** and **7** overview the opioid, mechanism of action, uses, safety issues, and focused monitoring.

COMMON NONOPIOID ANALGESICS

A multimodal approach is commonly used to treat pain in critically ill patients. Parental acetaminophen, parental ibuprofen, and enteral gabapentin are common nonopioid agents used to treat critically ill patents and used in the multimodal approach. Parental acetaminophen is an effective analgesic and antipyretic. Parental ibuprofen is a nonsteroidal antiinflammatory drug. Gapentinoids are anticonvulsant agents used for the management of neuropathic pain. **Table 2** provides an overview of these drugs, their purpose, and considerations in selecting these nonopioid analgesics.

Sedative Medications

Critically ill patients in the intensive care unit may require mechanical ventilation. A sedative analgesic is required to keep the patient comfortable and alleviate pain and agitation. Two common medications used are propofol and dexmedetomidine. These sedative analgesic drugs are overviewed in **Table 3**.

Case Report Regarding Benzodiazepine

LC is a 40-year-old man who is a construction worker. He fell 10 feet off a ladder and received several traumatic cervical fractures with the fall. His computed tomography scan was negative for a head injury and he is alert and oriented. He is

---

Box 6
Oxycodone

Oral semisynthetic opioid agonist analgesic.

Prototype is morphine.

Schedule II drug.

Mechanism of Action

Opioid agonist that binds with specific receptors in various sites of the central nervous system. Alters perception of pain and emotional response to pain. Onset is 10 to 15 minutes with peak in 30 to 60 minutes.

Uses

Enteral pain management for moderate to moderate severe pain. Available in sustained release tablet and oral solution.

Safety Issues

Black box warning

- Associated with life-threatening respiratory depression.
- High abuse potential.
- Concomitant use with warning for opioids with benzodiazepines or other central nervous system depressants may result in profound sedation, respiratory depression, coma, and death.

Safety alert

- Do not crush or chew sustained release form.

Focused Monitoring

- Central nervous system depression.
- Hepatotoxicity.
- Respiratory depression.

Data from Refs.[15,27,32]

---

in the trauma unit with a halo device to stabilize his cervical injuries. LC has a dilaudid patient-controlled anesthesia pump for pain management. LC is very anxious and agitated about his injuries, stating he needed to return to work, and would not be able to pay his bills. He expressed concern about his family with his loss of income. During LC's pain assessment, he asked for something to relax him and self-reported his pain was 3 of 10. The nurse found an as-needed order for lorazepam 2 to 4 mg intravenous for anxiety. The nurse decided to give LC lorazepam 4 mg intravenous for his agitation. Twenty minutes later, LC went into respiratory depression requiring naloxone administration. The nurse was unaware there is a black box warning for concomitant use of opioids with benzodiazepines because it can result in profound sedation, respiratory depression, coma, and death. The nurse's decision to use the lorazepam higher dose of 4 mg with the use of a dilaudid patient-controlled anesthesia pump was a poor decision that resulted in an incident report being written. Fortunately, the naloxone reversed the respiratory depression.

Box 7
Methadone

A long-acting synthetic opioid agonist.

Schedule II drug.

Available in oral, subcutaneous, intramuscular, and intravenous preparation.

Prototype is morphine.

Mechanism of Action

Synthetic opioid that is a central nervous system depression that causes sedation and respiratory depression.

Uses

Pain management for severe pain. Also used for detoxication treatment.

Safety Issues

Black box warning

- Respiratory depression and QT prolongation.
- Associated with abuse potential.
- Concomitant use with warning for opioids with benzodiazepines or other central nervous system depressants may result in profound sedation, respiratory depression, coma, and death.

Focused Monitoring

- Toxicity; naloxone is the antidote.
- Respiratory depression.
- Cardiac monitoring for QT interval prolongation and risk for Torsades de pointes.
- Close monitoring during treatment initiation and during dose titration owing to analgesic potency.

Data from Refs.[15,27,33]

Table 2
Nonopioid analgesics

Drug	Purpose	Considerations
Analgesic and antipyretic agent such as parenteral acetaminophen	Mild pain, and supplemental agent after surgery	Lacks antiplatelet effect and gastrointestinal toxicity Can cause hepatotoxicity
Nonsteroidal antiinflammatory drugs such as parenteral ibuprofen	Moderate acute pain and febrile condition	Can worsen renal insufficiency, gastrointestinal bleeding, and platelet dysfunction
Gabapentinoids such as gabapentin	Management of neuropathic pain	Requires enteral administration Can cause sedation, dizziness, and ataxia

Data from Refs.[15,25,27,34]

Table 3 Sedative medications		
Drug	**Purpose**	**Consideration**
Propofol	Potent sedative-hypnotic Mechanical ventilated patients	Infusion is titratable to desired depth of sedation Immediate onset Rapid awakening with discontinuation
Dexmedetomidine	Effective sedative sympatholytic with moderate anxiolysis and analgesia Mechanically ventilated patients	No significant effect on respiratory drive Depth of sedation keeps patient comfortable while allowing patient to be easily awakened and interactive

Data from Pandharipande P, Parsons P, Finlay G, editors. Pain control in the critically ill adult patient. Available at: www.uptodate.com. Accessed April 26, 2017.

SUMMARY

Acute pain is a universal pervasive source of distress in the critically ill patient. Serious life-threatening or fatal respiratory depression may occur with pharmacologic intervention with sedative analgesics such as morphine, fentanyl, and hydromorphone. The nurse has an ethical and legal duty to provide safe, quality, and accountable pain management. The nurse must apply critical thinking and clinical reasoning skills in the administration of pain medications in a critically ill patient to prevent serious side effects and adverse reactions. The nurse needs to acquire self-efficacy in conducting a comprehensive pain assessment in a verbal and nonverbal patient and monitoring the patient's response to the pharmacologic intervention. This article presented a toolkit for pain management that discussed

Table 4 Benzodiazepines		
Drug	**Purpose**	**Consideration**
Midazolam (Versed)	Potent amnestic and anxiolytic agent Anesthesia, procedural sedation, agitation	Works on central nervous system to cause sedation, muscle relaxation, short term memory loss, and reduce anxiety Half-life may be prolonged in critically ill patients
Lorazepam (Ativan)	Sedative, amnestic, anti-convulsant properties	Delayed onset and accumulation in peripheral tissues Risk of oversedation Risk of delirium Intermittent bolus dosing preferred
Diazepam (Valium)	Potent sedative and muscle relaxant effects Patients at risk for alcohol withdrawal and/or seizures	Rapid onset May accumulate and cause prolonged sedation Risk of delirium

Data from Pandharipande P, Parsons P, Finlay G, editors. Pain control in the critically ill adult patient. Available at: www.uptodate.com. Accessed April 26, 2017; and Wilson B, Shannon M, Shields K. Pearson nurse's drug guide 2016. Hoboken (NJ): Pearson Education Inc; 2016.

Table 5
Antipsychotics

Drug	Purpose	Consideration
Haloperidol (Haldol)	Moderately sedating antipsychotic used to treat hyperactivity of delirium and ICU psychosis Agitation Adjunctive treatment of alcohol and opioid withdrawal	Interferes with metabolism of common intensive care drugs and can prolong the QT wave Hypotension
Olanzapine (Zyprexa)	Potential as needed adjunct to haloperidol for delirium and agitation Available as a short-acting IM agent	Orthostatic hypotension Somnolence Anticholinergic effects Prolonged QT wave
Quetiapine (Seroquel)	Potential as-needed adjunct to haloperidol Sedative effect	Requires enteral route of administration

Abbreviations: ICU, intensive care unit; IM, intramuscularly.
Data from Pandharipande P, Parsons P, Finlay G, editors. Pain control in the critically ill adult patient. Available at: www.uptodate.com. Accessed April 26, 2017; and Wilson B, Shannon M, Shields K. Pearson nurse's drug guide 2016. Hoboken (NJ): Pearson Education Inc; 2016.

the need for the nurse to embrace an ethical framework, and incorporate pain management guidelines that included the Joint Commission, Medicare, and national nursing organizations into their plan of care. Pharmacologic interventions were presented that included common intravenous sedative analgesics, oral opioids, nonopioid analgesics, sedative medications, benzodiazepines (**Table 4**), and antipsychotics (**Table 5**). Case reports were presented involving special populations to apply clinical reasoning skills learned in this pain pharmacologic intervention article.

REFERENCES

1. American Nurses Association and American Society for Pain Management Nursing. Pain management nursing: scope and standards of practice, 2nd edition. Silver Spring (MD): 2016.

2. Lome B. Acute pain and the critically ill trauma patient. Crit Care Nurs Q 2005; 28(2):200–7.

3. U.S. Department of Health and Human Services (HHS), Office of the Surgeon General. Facing addition in America: the Surgeon General's report on Alcohol, drugs, and health. Chapter 1 Introduction and overview of the report. Washington, DC: HHS; 2016. p. 1–26.

4. Prescription Drug Monitoring Program Training and Technical Assistance Center. Prescription drug monitoring frequently asked question (FAQ). Available at: www. pdmpassist.org. Accessed March 10, 2017.

5. Doody Q, Noonan M. Nursing research ethics, guidance and application in practice. Br J Nurs 2016;25(14):803–7.

6. Joint Commission. Joint commission statement of pain management. Available at: http://www.jointcommision.org/joint_commission__statement_on_pain_manage ment/. Accessed March 10, 2017.

7. Joint Commission on Accreditation of Healthcare Organization. Joint commission on accreditation of healthcare organizations pain standards for 2001. Available at: http://www.jacaho.com/standard/pm.html. Accessed March 10, 2017.

8. The Joint Commission E-dition. Joint commission FAQ page. Available at: https://www.jointcommission.org/about/jointcommisionfaq.aspx?Categoryid=58#2493. Accessed March 10, 2017.

9. Baker D. History of the Joint Commission's. Pain standard lessons for today's prescription opioid epidemic. J Am Med Assoc 2017;317(11):117–8.

10. The Joint Commission. Proposed acute pin assessment and management standards hospital accreditation program. 1–3. Public Comment. 2017. Available at: www.jointcommission.org/assets.1/6/2017_Draft_Pain_Standards.pdf. Accessed March 10, 2017.

11. HCAHPS fact sheet. Baltimore (MD): Centers for Medicare & Medicaid Services (CMC); 2015. p. 1–4. Available at: http://www.hcahpsononline.org/Facts.aspx. Accessed March 10, 2017.

12. Hospitals & Health Networks. Doctors urge CMS, Joint commission to rethink pain treatment to help stem opioid epidemic. Physicians for Responsible Opioid Prescribing petition for rule making. 2016. Available at: http://www.heahpsonline.org. Accessed March 10, 2017.

13. Centers & Medicaid Services. HCAHPS Survey. 2017. Available at: http://www.heahpsonline.org. Accessed March 10, 2017.

14. Department of Health & Human Services. Cavanaugh S. Letter response to Physicians for Responsible Opioid Prescribing petition. 2016. Available at: http://www.heahpsonline.org. Accessed March 10, 2017.

15. Pandharipande P, Parsons P, Finlay G, editors. Pain control in the critically ill adult patient. Available at: www.uptodate.com. Accessed April 26, 2017.

16. Rose L, Simth O, Gelinas C, et al. Critical care nurses' pain assessment and management practices: a survey in Canada. Am J Crit Care 2012;21(4):251–60.

17. Haslam L, Dale C, Knechtel L, et al. Pain descriptors for critically ill patients unable to self-report. J Adv Nurs 2011;68(5):1082–9.

18. Puntillo K. Pain assessment and management in the critically ill: wizardry or science? Am J Nurs 2003;12(4):310–6.

19. Chanques G, Jaber S, Barbotte E, et al. Impact of systematic evaluation of pain and agitation in the intensive care unit. Crit Care Med 2006;34(6):1691–9.

20. Rijkenberg S, Stilma W, Endeman H, et al. Pain measurement in mechanically ventilated critically ill patients: behavioral pain scale versus critical-care pain observation tool. J Crit Care 2015;30:167–72.

21. Arbour C, Gelinas C. Setting goals for pain management when using a behavioral scale: example with the critical-care pain observation tool. Crit Care Nurse 2011;31(6):66–8.

22. Drew D, Gordan D, Morgan B, et al. The use of as-needed range orders for opioid analgesics in the management of pain: a consensus statement of the American society of pain management nurses and the American pain society pain management nursing. 2014. Available at: http://www.aspmn.org/documents/RangeOrderPublished2014.pdf. Accessed April 26, 2017.

23. Hayes K, Gordon DB. Delivering quality pain management: the challenge for nurses. AORN J 2015;101:328–34. Available at: https://www.aorn.org/websitedata/ceararticle/pdf_file/CEA15508-0001.pdf. Accessed April 15, 2017.

24. Truven health analytics dyamed plus. Morphine Sulfate. Available at: http://www. dynamed.com/login.aspx?direct=true&site=DynaMed&id=233078.   Accessed April 26, 2017.
25. Tietze K, Fuchs, B, Parsons P, et al, editors. Sedative-analgesic medications in critically ill adults: properties, dosage, regimens, and adverse effects. Available at: www.uptodate.com. Accessed April 26, 2017.
26. Morphine: drug information. Available at: www.uptodate.com. Accessed April 26, 2017.
27. Wilson B, Shannon M, Shields K. Pearson nurse's drug guide 2016. Hoboken (NJ): Pearson Education Inc; 2016.
28. Truven health analytics dyamed plus. Fentanyl. Available at: http://www. dynamed.com/login.aspx?direct=true&site=DynaMed&id=233078.   Accessed April 26, 2017.
29. Fentanyl: drug information. Available at: www.uptodate.com. Accessed April 26, 2017.
30. Truven health analytics dyamed plus hydromorphone. Available at: http://www. dynamed.com/login.aspx?direct=true&site=DynaMed&id=233043.   Accessed April 26, 2017.
31. Hydromorphone: drug information. Available at: www.uptodate.com. Accessed April 26, 2017.
32. Truven health analytics dyamed plus. Oxycodone. Available at: http://www. dynamed.com/login.aspx?direct=true&site=DynaMed&id=233077.   Accessed April 26, 2017.
33. Truven health analytics dyamed plus. Methadone. Available at: http://www. dynamed.com/login.aspx?direct=true&site=DynaMed&id=233079.   Accessed April 26, 2017.
34. Truven health analytics dyamed plus. Gabapentin. Available at: http://www. dynamed.com/login.aspx?direct=true&site=DynaMed&id=233455.   Accessed April 26, 2017.

Pain and Complementary Therapies

Amy S. Hamlin, PhD, MSN, FNP-BC, APRN*, T. Michelle Robertson, DNP, FNP-BC, APRN

KEYWORDS

- Pain • Complementary and alternative therapy (CAT) • Relaxation breathing
- Acupuncture • Acupressure • Guided imagery • Music therapy • Aromatherapy

KEY POINTS

- A large percentage of the population affected by painful conditions/diseases.
- Complementary and alternative therapies (CATs) are being increasingly used and requested by patients in pain.
- Evidence-based practice supports the use of CATs as a part of the treatment plan for patients with both acute and chronic pain.
- Nurses are well placed to implement various CAT modalities.

INTRODUCTION

Complementary and alternative therapy (CAT) is a term used for practices and therapies that may not be part of the standard medical treatment plan. The terms complementary and alternative, although often used interchangeably, are different. Complementary medicine or complementary therapies are those used as an adjunct to, or together with, traditional therapies. Alternative medicine or alternative therapies are used in place of traditional treatments. The use of complementary therapies dates back in nursing to Florence Nightingale. Her historical accounts of holistic nursing care include the use of heat, massage, music, and touch. Nursing education has long incorporated concepts and components of CAT in the nursing plan of care. The National Center for Complementary and Integrative Health lists the 10 most common complementary health approaches used among adults as natural products (dietary supplements), deep breathing, yoga and other exercises, chiropractic, meditation, special diets, homeopathy, relaxation, and guided imagery.[1]

Pain

The International Association for the Study of Pain defines pain as, "...an unpleasant sensory and emotional experience associated with actual or potential tissue

Disclosure: The authors have nothing to disclose.
Austin Peay State University School of Nursing, PO Box 4658, Clarksville, TN 37044, USA
* Corresponding author.
E-mail address: hamlina@apsu.edu

damage or described in terms of such damage."[2] Pain is separated into categories of acute and chronic. Acute pain occurs suddenly and is described in qualitative words such as sharp or stabbing. Acute pain is commonly the result of something specific such as an injury, and it lasts for 6 months or less. Chronic pain is an ongoing complaint of pain that lasts for 3 to 6 months or longer.[3] In contrast with acute pain, it is often described with terms such as dull, throbbing, pressure, or burning. Chronic pain can occur after an injury is long healed or in conditions in which no known injury occurred. The National Center for Complementary and Integrative Health lists the top 10 diseases and conditions for which complementary therapies are used among adults as back pain, neck pain, joint pain, joint stiffness, cardiovascular conditions, arthritis, fibromyalgia, anxiety, and depression.[4]

Prevalence of Pain and Complementary and Alternative Therapy Usage

The prevalence of pain can be difficult to quantify based on the varying subjective accounts of what pain is to the individual. The US Department of Health and Human Services indicates that pain affects more Americans than heart disease, cancer, and diabetes combined.[5] The National Center for Health Statistics estimates that 1 in every 4 Americans has pain lasting longer than 24 hours.[5] Research shows 25 million American adults have daily pain.[6] The National Health Interview Survey found that half of American adults (125 million) had pain that was identified as musculoskeletal. More than 40% of those adults used a complementary approach in treating the musculoskeletal pain. The overall out-of-pocket expenditure for complementary health approaches is approximately $30 billion per year.[7]

The Role of Nurses

Patients are increasingly knowledgeable that CATs are available to them; however, not all patients have specific knowledge of the different complementary therapies and how they may be incorporated into the treatment plan. It is the responsibility of nurses to be holistic in their approach to pain control and be open-minded to the integration of complementary modalities. Alternative medicine or complementary therapies may be sought out by the patient for various reasons. Medications for pain may be too expensive or not covered fully by insurance, or the patient may think that the medications are ineffective for pain management. In addition, some patients fear that they may become addicted to medications if they start taking them. There are many reasons why a patient may choose alternative and complementary therapies.

When considering using CAT for patient care, nurses must first complete a comprehensive patient history and physical assessment. It is important that nurses complete a pain assessment tool that is specific to the patient population (eg, infants, pediatrics, adults, and elderly, nonresponsive, sedated). Nurses must ensure that the tool used has high validity and reliability. It is critical to obtain a detailed medication history to include all over-the-counter treatments and natural/herbal supplements. A holistic plan of care cannot be established without first discussing the patient's personal goals for pain management and integrating cultural/ethnic/religious variables and values. The nurse and patient must work collaboratively to establish short-term and long-term goals for patient pain. The plan of care should include an interdisciplinary approach for best outcomes.[8] **Table 1** provides a summary of evidence-based complementary therapies that may be used by qualified nurses working in acute and critical care settings.

Table 1 Examples of complementary therapies	
Complementary Therapy Category	**Examples of Treatments**
Body-based methods	Touch Acupressure Massage Acupuncture Yoga
Energy therapies	Therapeutic touch Reiki Electromagnetic therapy Qigong
Diet and herbal preparations	Dietary supplements Botanicals (herbal preparations) Diet/nutrition Probiotics
Mind therapies	Meditation Relaxation Relaxed breathing Guided imagery Hypnosis
Sensory therapies	Aromatherapy Music therapy
Movement therapies	Pilates Dance therapy

COMPLEMENTARY THERAPIES AND PAIN MANAGEMENT

Treatment of both acute and chronic pain typically involves a combination of pharmacologic and provider-based interventions. Although this may be effective for some patients, it may not be for others. Pain medications can be ineffective and inadequate in controlling acute or chronic pain. Use of pain medications, especially with repeated and frequent usage, involves the risk of adverse reactions, overuse, and dependency. Some patients do not desire a pharmacologic course of therapy. Others may report that pain medications are ineffective in managing their pain, or they may be experiencing adverse or undesirable side effects.

When pain control cannot be reached at a satisfactory level, or the patient requests an alternative or modified treatment plan, it is appropriate to consider the implementation of complementary therapies. There are many evidence-based CAT methods that have shown effectiveness in the management of acute and chronic pain. Complementary therapies have been shown not only to decrease the pain experience but also to enhance patient functioning and quality of life. **Table 2** describes specific complementary therapies that can be used as adjunct therapies in the management of various pain conditions.

Although CAT therapies are shown in the literature to decrease pain, improve function, and improve the overall quality of life, they are not always implemented consistently. Research shows that even though nurses are aware and educated about CAT therapies, they are unsure of the effectiveness of the impact on pain and unclear about specific CAT techniques or how to perform them.[9] This uncertainty is seen as a clear barrier to evidence-based practice.

Table 2
Complementary therapies and pain management

Complementary Therapy	Effect on the Body	Conditions Responsive to Identified CAT
Relaxation breathing	Releasing tension in the body through controlled breathing	Procedural pain, fibromyalgia, chronic pain, burn pain, labor pain, TMJ dysfunction
Essential oils and aromatherapy	Signal transmitted via olfactory bulb causing serotonin, endorphin, and noradrenaline release	Osteoarthritis, posttonsillectomy pain, postarthroscopy pain, post–breast biopsy pain, swollen joints, muscular pain, rheumatoid arthritis
Music therapy	Relaxation replaces tension and worry, distracting attention away from pain	Physical rehabilitation, procedural pain, burn debridement, cancer pain, labor pain, palliative care, postoperative pain, neuropathic pain
Guided imagery	Relaxation and distraction refocusing pain perception	Fibromyalgia, sickle cell pain, procedural pain, postoperative pain, chronic pain, low back pain, cancer pain, headaches, burn pain, arthritis
Acupuncture	Stimulation of endorphin release enhancing natural pain killer cells	Back and neck pain, renal colic, postoperative pain, knee pain, migraine headaches, facial pain, osteoarthritis, rheumatoid arthritis, sciatica, dysmenorrhea
Acupressure	Induction of relaxation, distraction of the nervous system, and activation of natural pain killer cells	Minor trauma pain, dysmenorrhea, chronic headaches, low back pain, neck pain, labor pain, chronic pain

Abbreviation: TMJ, temporomandibular joint.
Data from Refs.[14–16,22–29,31,32,34–43]

Legal Issues and the Nurse Practice Act

Patients may ask nurses to perform or participate in various complementary or alternative interventions. It is the nurse's responsibility to assess whether the intervention is appropriate and whether there are any potential risks to the patient. In addition, to perform CATs, nurses must have the appropriate education, skills, and credentials required for the specific technique.[10]

There is no national standard for implementation of CATs. Nurses are responsible for knowing the laws of their particular states, as outlined in the Nurse Practice Act. Keep in mind that not all 50 states address or provide guidelines related to nurses and the implementation of CATs.

ESSENTIAL OILS AND AROMATHERAPY

The use of essential oils and aromatherapy are two complementary therapies dating back thousands of years. These therapies, the fastest growing CATs, are popular and readily available to patients to purchase at their local markets or health food stores. Essential oils and aromatherapy products may not be readily available in hospitals or other health care settings, and nurses may have limited training or knowledge on their use.

Essential oils are made from various parts of plants, herbs, or trees (ie, bark, stem, flower, rind, and root), and are used for various therapeutic reasons by patients from all cultures and backgrounds. There are many varieties of essential oils, and their indications are extensive. Essential oils may be used topically, diffused through the air, inhaled, or added to liquid or food for oral ingestion. They may be incorporated with other CAT modalities, including massage therapy. Essential oils have the ability to prevent bacterial and fungal growth, support wound healing, prevent or decrease inflammation, and provide comfort, and they possess both anesthetic and analgesic properties.[11,12]

Aromatherapy comprises the use of fragrant essential oils for various healing and health benefits. Aromatherapy is very effective when used as an adjunctive therapy for pain management.[11,12] Once the essential oil is absorbed into the circulatory and nervous systems, it is thought that all body systems can be affected by the aromatherapy,[13] and this is important to consider when developing a treatment plan specific to pain.

With regard to pain, various studies connect the use of aromatherapy and essential oils with pain control. The most commonly studied essential oil showing analgesic effects is lavender. Studies have shown that lavender is associated with decreased pain levels in patients after cesareans, after tonsillectomy, after operative arthroscopic knee surgery, and after breast biopsy.[14–16] Other essential oils assisting with pain management include German chamomile, sweet marjoram, dwarf pine, rosemary, and ginger.[17] These oils have shown improved pain management and increased comfort in patients with rheumatoid arthritis, headaches, muscular pain, swollen joints, and other pain complaints. Combining aromatherapy with massage has been found to increase the efficacy of pain management.[18,19]

When considering the use of essential oils as a part of the plan of care, nurses must take into account potential risks, implications, demonstrated efficacy, and indications for the therapy. Typically, essential oils should not be used at 100% concentration. They need to be diluted to a lower concentration, especially for patients less than 2 years old.[11] Essential oils can have adverse effects, including risk for toxicity, skin irritation, photosensitivity, and severe allergic reactions. If there is suspicion for potential allergic reaction, skin testing may need to be performed before use. Proper dilution minimizes risks of reaction and sensitivity.[20]

Essential oils and aromatherapy products are not regulated by the US Food and Drug Administration (FDA). Only essential oils and products that are unaltered and sold from reputable companies who do not adulterate the products should be used.[11] Nurses should not administer essential oils without proper education and a well-developed protocol. If used in a hospital or outpatient setting, material safety data sheets describing the oil's properties and ingredients should be available.

Essential oils and aromatherapy should be used cautiously with pregnant women or women who are breastfeeding. Some essential oils should be avoided because of risks in infants, young children, and elderly patients.

MUSIC THERAPY

Music therapy is a complementary sensory therapy that has been used by various cultures for thousands of years. Music therapy involves listening to music, writing music, or playing music. The most common form of music therapy involves actively listening to music. Patients can wear headphones or listen through speakers. They may choose their music or listen to a prescribed playlist developed by a music therapist. From classical music to nature sounds, and country to rock and roll, music can have distinct physical effects, including decreased anxiety and stress, improved mood, decreased heart rate and blood pressure, increased circulation, and decreased pain perception.[21]

Research has shown that music therapy has a positive impact on the pain experience. Reduced pain levels, lessened muscle tension, and decreased opioid use have been observed in obstetric patients in labor participating in music therapy.[22] Other diagnoses or conditions in which music therapy shows efficacy include patients with neuropathic pain, cancer pain, pain associated with burn debridement, procedural pain, postoperative pain, and pain related to palliative care.[22–24]

Music therapy can be initiated in any patient care setting. Multiple studies show significant differences in pain levels of patients in hospitals, intensive care units, palliative care areas, and postoperative settings. Music therapy may be implemented by a trained music therapist, but it may also be independently initiated by the nurse, patient, family member, or any other member of the health care team.[21] To facilitate music therapy, nurses should encourage the patient or family to bring listening equipment (eg, iPod, MP3 player, compact discs, radio) or access available listening materials through the health care facility. If proper equipment is available, there is no cost for this therapy, and there are minimal to no potential adverse side effects.

Research has shown that environmental manipulation and patient involvement increase the efficacy of music therapy when used for pain management. Allowing patients to self-select their preferred styles of music has shown value-added outcomes.[24] In addition, making adjustments to the patient's environment, such as dimming the lights, providing a blanket, turning off electronics and cell phones, and putting up a do-not-disturb sign, have increased overall effectiveness.[24]

GUIDED IMAGERY

Guided imagery is a cognitive therapy focused on conjuring pleasant images in the patient's mind, with the goal of promoting relaxation and symptom relief. The therapy assists the patient to concentrate on mental images, scenes, or pictures during a period of relaxation. Patients may imagine themselves on a warm beach or at an amusement park, or they may envision their bodies fighting a specific disease process. All 5 senses should be involved in the experience. Patients should imagine a scenario in which they can hear, smell, feel, taste, and touch. Guided imagery should not be confused with hypnosis because there is no induction of a trancelike state, and patients are not expected to respond to requests of the person performing the guided imagery.[25]

Guided imagery is one of the most straightforward complementary therapies to implement. It is usually performed over a period of 10 to 20 minutes, and is convenient, noninvasive, and has limited risk of adverse effects. Guided imagery can be completed in any patient care setting or in the patient's home. It is without any real cost. It can be implemented by any nurse or caregiver trained in guided imagery technique. Prerecorded scripts may be used as a model or patients may self-lead their therapy.[26]

It is thought that guided imagery works to lessen the pain experience by decreasing the sensory and emotional aspects of pain.[27] Throughout the guided imagery process, the patient is calmed, and relaxation occurs, allowing the body and mind to reach a peaceful state, ultimately releasing the emotional distress caused by pain. Pain is relieved through distraction achieved through the guided imagery process. Patients can shift their focus from feelings of discomfort to feelings of contentment and enjoyment.[28]

Evidence shows that guided imagery decreases pain levels in patients with various diagnoses and conditions, including patients with pain from fibromyalgia, sickle cell disease, cancer, headaches, burns, and arthritis.[25–28] Guided imagery has also been successfully implemented in patients experiencing procedural, postoperative, chronic, and low back pain.[25–28] Guided imagery should not be used on all patients. It should be avoided in patients who are disoriented, have dementia or delirium, are actively psychotic, or who cannot distinguish imagined images from what is real. In addition, patients unable to hear or those who cannot verbally communicate may not be candidates for guided imagery.[28]

ACUPUNCTURE

It is thought that the ritual of acupuncture has existed for centuries. The practice of acupuncture dates back to ancient Chinese customs and has grown in prevalence in the United States since the 1970s. In 1997, the National Institutes of Health (NIH) documented the efficacy and safety of acupuncture. Acupuncture is used in a variety of health care settings, including both inpatient and outpatient areas. The therapy is covered by some insurance policies when it is determined to be medically necessary.

Acupuncture is typically performed by inserting sterile thin needles under the skin to stimulate acupoints along pathways called meridians. It is thought that the acupoints block the flow of a person's qi (chi), or the movement of energy. The process of acupuncture allows the release of the blocked qi, evoking the body's ability to heal itself.

There are variations to traditional acupuncture that patients may choose to explore. Electroacupuncture involves attaching the acupuncture needles to an electrical current as a means to further stimulate the acupoints. Laser acupuncture, a newer method, is a noninvasive alternative that has shown improved efficacy in certain conditions, including musculoskeletal pain. It is unknown whether traditional acupuncture, electroacupuncture, or laser acupuncture is more effective than the others.[29]

Acupuncture is widely used for a variety of medical conditions, including both acute and chronic pain. Research has shown acupuncture to have analgesic effects similar to those of pharmacologic interventions.[30] Patients using acupuncture as a complementary therapy frequently report overall pain reduction and improved quality of life. It is thought that acupuncture relieves pain through the release of endorphins, the body's natural pain killer hormones.[31] Clinical studies have shown acupuncture as being effective in the treatment of back and neck pain, knee pain, migraine headaches, dysmenorrhea, facial pain, osteoarthritis, postoperative pain, sciatica, renal colic, and rheumatoid arthritis.[29,31,32]

Not all patients are candidates for acupuncture. Patients with neutropenia, thrombocytopenia, or coagulopathy, or those taking anticoagulant/antiplatelet medications, should not receive acupuncture therapy. Acupuncture should not be performed on limbs with lymphedema or over the site of a tumor or metastasis. It is thought that acupuncture may stimulate labor, so caution is needed when considering acupuncture for pregnant women. Patients with pacemakers should not use electroacupuncture because it is associated with electrical currents.[33]

Acupuncture does not come under the standard scope of practice for registered nurses, and a separate licensure is required in most states. Nurses should not perform acupuncture without appropriate training, certification, and credentials. Individual states regulate the practice of acupuncture, and each state has different laws.

ACUPRESSURE

Acupressure, like acupuncture, is an ancient practice focused on releasing and stimulating qi from acupoints along meridians of the body. Acupressure is often referred to as needleless acupuncture. The technique differs from acupuncture in that the practitioner's fingers and hands are used, instead of needles and lasers, to apply pressure over the acupoints. The practice is noninvasive, nonpainful, and inexpensive. It can be performed in any patient care setting, and there are few potential adverse effects. Patients can also be taught various acupressure procedures, allowing them to be self-reliant and in charge of their care.

Acupressure has been shown to be effective in treating pain, including minor trauma pain, dysmenorrhea, chronic headache, low back, neck, labor, and chronic pain.[34–40] Auricular point acupressure, a specific type of acupressure targeting acupoints along the outer ear, has shown improved functioning and pain relief in patients with chronic low back pain and cancer-related pain.[34,36]

Any practitioner performing acupressure must have training in acupressure techniques and must be cautious when using acupressure on frail, elderly, or very young patients.[35] As identified earlier with acupuncture, nurses must check with their individual state boards of nursing to assess the nursing scope of practice related to this complementary therapy.

RELAXATION BREATHING

Managing pain is an ongoing challenge for patients and nurses. When a person is in pain, there are both physiologic and psychological reactions. Relaxation breathing is a mind-body modality that combines slow, deep breathing with relaxation. In order to perform relaxation breathing, the patient is instructed to take slow, deep, even breaths while relaxing the body. The patient may be in a sitting position or lying down, and should be instructed to breathe deeply from the abdomen.

Relaxation breathing has shown lessened intensity and emotional reaction in patients reporting pain. Deep breathing increases bronchopulmonary afferent nerve communication with the central nervous system, and relaxation promotes parasympathetic activity while decreasing the activation of the sympathetic nervous system. This process results in deactivation of the sympathetic nervous system, reducing the body's overall state of stress and excitability, and improving the patient's sense of well-being.[41]

Relaxation breathing has been shown to be a beneficial intervention when used by patients in various states of pain with a range of diagnoses and conditions. Participation in relaxation breathing has been associated with decreased pain in patients with burns, especially when implemented during painful dressing changes.[41] Overall pain reduction has been associated with female patients with fibromyalgia when exposed to relaxation breathing, specifically when slow breathing techniques were used.[42] Alternative diagnoses and conditions in which relaxation breathing may be helpful include procedural pain, labor pain, and temporomandibular joint dysfunction. With regard to chronic pain, use of relaxation breathing in combination with other CAT modalities such as yoga, qigong, and tai chi has been associated with higher pain thresholds. Note that deep breathing techniques without the relaxation component have been shown to be ineffective in reducing reported pain levels.[43]

Advantages of relaxation breathing include no cost, simplicity of implementation, and minimal risk of adverse effects. There is no required timing for relaxation breathing. It can be implemented over a period of a few minutes and last as long as the patient wants to continue. Nurses may apply this modality into the plan of care without any specific training or education. Relaxation breathing can be implemented in all health care settings as well as in the patient's home.

In rare instances, patients participating in relaxation breathing report increased anxiety, unpleasant thoughts, and feelings of loss of control. Patients with epilepsy, a history of abuse or trauma, and certain psychiatric conditions may have an exacerbation of symptoms or increased anxiety when participating in relaxation techniques.[44]

SUMMARY

When a patient experiences pain it can have an adverse impact on physiologic and psychological processes. To provide holistic care, nurses must recruit all measures necessary to help meet the patient-centered goals. Knowledge of CATs can provide nurses with valuable resources/interventions to improve patients' painful conditions or diseases. Nurses can incorporate nonpharmacologic CAT interventions in hospitals, outpatient settings, or in patients' homes. CATs are overall inexpensive, easy to implement, present minimal side effects, and are evidence based when used for pain in identified diagnoses and conditions. **Box 1** describes the nursing responsibilities and questions that must be asked when considering implementation of complementary therapies.[45]

There are multiple resources available to explore all aspects of CATs. The American Holistic Nurses Association provides information about various complementary therapies, including position statements and information about education, training, certifications, and endorsements. The Web site also has a link addressing the Nurse Practice Acts by individual state. Ultimately, it is the responsibility of nurses to understand the rules and regulations of their states and the policies and procedures of the facility or organization in which they are employed.

Box 1
Complementary and alternative therapies and nursing responsibilities

Appropriateness of the complementary therapy:

- Is the CAT evidence based?
- Will the CAT meet the patient goals for pain control?
- What is the anticipated effect of the selected CAT?
- Are there any potential risks to the patient?
- Is the patient informed and has consent been verified?
- Was adequate assessment performed to justify full benefits and risks?

Required knowledge, skill, and education:

- Does the nurse have education, training, or certification required to perform the CAT?
- Has the nurse followed the laws and guidelines identified in the state Nurse Practice Act and the policy/procedure manual of the employer?

Data from Complementary therapies. College of Nurses of Ontario. Available at: https://www.cno.org/globalassets/docs/prac/41021_comptherapies.pdf. Accessed March 24, 2017.

REFERENCES

1. Use of complementary health approaches in the U.S. 10 most common complementary health approaches among adults-2012. National Center for Complementary and Integrative health. Available at: https://nccih.nih.gov/file/3039. Accessed April 24, 2017.
2. IASP taxonomy. International Association for the Study of Pain. Available at: http://www.iasp-pain.org/Taxonomy. Accessed April 24, 2017.
3. Chronic pain syndrome: what is a chronic pain syndrome? Institute of Chronic Pain. Available at: http://www.instituteforchronicpain.org/understanding-chronic-pain/what-is-chronic-pain/chronic-pain-syndrome. Accessed April 20, 2017.
4. Diseases/conditions for which complementary health approaches are most frequently used among adults- 2012. National Center for Complementary and Integrative Health. Available at: https://nccih.nih.gov/file/2979. Accessed April 10, 2017.
5. Research portfolio online reporting tools. Pain management. US Department of Health and Human Services. Available at: https://report.nih.gov/nihfactsheets/ViewFactSheet.aspx?csid=57. Accessed April 10, 2017.
6. Nahin RL. Estimates of pain prevalence and severity in adults: United States, 2012. J Pain 2015;16(8):769–80.
7. Clark TC, Black LI, Stussman BJ, et al. Trends in the use of complementary health approaches among adults: United States, 2002-2012. Natl Health Stat Rep 2015; 19:1–16.
8. Delgado R, York A, Lee C, et al. Assessing the quality, efficacy, and effectiveness of the current evidence base of active self-care complementary and integrative medicine therapies for the management of chronic pain: a rapid evidence assessment of the literature. Pain Med 2014;15(Suppl 1):S9–20.
9. Gruber BNC. Side effects of complementary and alternative medicine. Allergy 2003;53:707–16.
10. What is a holistic nursing? American Holistic Nurses Association. Available at: http://www.ahna.org/. Accessed March 11, 2017.
11. Allard ME, Katseres J. Using essential oils to enhance nursing practice and for self-care. Am J Nurs 2016;116(2):42–9.
12. Jopke K, Sanders H, White-Traut R. Use of essential oils following traumatic burn injury: a case study. J Pediatr Nurs 2017;34:72–7.
13. Halcon L. Aromatherapy. In: Lindquist R, editor. Complementary and alternative therapies in nursing. 7th edition. New York: Springer; 2014. p. 323–44.
14. Thomas D. Aromatherapy: mythical, magical, or medicinal? Holist Nurs Pract 2002;17(1):8–16.
15. Huang S-H, Fang L, Fang S-H. The effectiveness of aromatherapy with lavender essential oil in relieving post arthroscopy pain. JMED Res 2014. http://dx.doi.org/10.5171/2014.183395.
16. Soltani R, Soheilipour S, Hajhashemi V, et al. Evaluation of the effect of aromatherapy with lavender essential oil on post-tonsillectomy pain in pediatric patients: a randomized controlled trial. Int J Pediatr Otorhinolaryngol 2013; 77(9):1579–81.
17. Ali B, Al-Wabel A, Shams S, et al. Essential oils used in aromatherapy: a systemic review. Asian Pac J Trop Biomed 2015;5(8):601–11.
18. Metin ZG, Ozdemir L. The effects of aromatherapy massage and reflexology on pain and fatigue in patients with rheumatoid arthritis: a randomized control trial. Pain Manag Nurs 2016;17(2):140–9.

19. Nasiri A, Mahmodi MA, Nobakht Z. Effect of aromatherapy massage with lavender essential oil on pain in patients with osteoarthritis of the knee: a randomized controlled clinical trial. Complement Ther Clin Pract 2016;25:75–80.

20. Peterson D. Indications and contraindications for aromatherapy. ARC Newsletter 2012;18:1–4.

21. Colwell CM, Edwards R, Hernandez E, et al. Impact of music therapy interventions (listening, composition, Orff-based) on the physiological and psychosocial behaviors of hospitalized children: a feasibility study. J Pediatr Nurs 2013;28: 249–57.

22. Cole LC, LoBiondo-Wood G. Music as an adjuvant therapy in control of pain and symptoms in hospitalized adults: a systematic review. Pain Manag Nurs 2014; 15(1):406–25.

23. Korhan EA, Uyar M, Eyigor C, et al. The effects of music therapy on pain in patients with neuropathic pain. Pain Manag Nurs 2012;15(1):306–14.

24. Gutsgell KJ, Schluchter M, Margevicius S, et al. Music therapy reduces pain in palliative care patients: a randomized controlled trial. J Pain Symptom Manage 2013;45(5):822–31.

25. Burnett J. Guided imagery as an adjunct to pharmacological pain control at end of life. North American Association of Christians in Social Work. Available at: http://www.nacsw.org/Publications/Proceedings2012/BurnettJGuidedImagery.pdf. Accessed April 10, 2017.

26. Lewandowski W, Good M, Draucker CB. Changes in the meaning of pain with the use of guided imagery. Pain Manag Nurs 2005;6(2):58–67.

27. Ling Y, Francis JP. Relaxation and imagery for chronic pain, nonmalignant pain: effects on pain symptoms, quality of life, and mental health. Pain Manag Nurs 2010;11(3):159–68.

28. Burhenn P, Olausson J, Villegas G, et al. Guided imagery for pain control. Clin J Oncol Nurs 2014;18(5):501–3.

29. Hinman R, McCrory P, Pirotta M, et al. Acupuncture for chronic knee pain: a randomized clinical trial. JAMA 2014;312(13):1313–22.

30. Lee H, Lee J-H, Choi M, et al. Acupuncture for acute low back pain: a systematic review. Clin J Pain 2013;29(2):172–85.

31. Liu L, Skinner M, McDonough S, et al. Acupuncture for low back pain: an overview of systematic reviews. Evid Based Complement Alternat Med 2015;2015: 328196.

32. Acupuncture: in depth. National Center for Integrative and Complementary Health. Available at: https://nccih.nih.gov/health/acupuncture/introduction. Accessed February 27, 2017.

33. Acupuncture. Mayo Clinic. Available at: http://www.mayoclinic.org/tests-procedures/acupuncture/basics/risks/prc-20020778. Accessed March 11, 2017.

34. Lin W-C, Yeh CH, Chien L-C, et al. The anti-inflammatory actions of auricular point acupressure for chronic low back pain. Evid Based Complement Alternat Med 2015. http://dx.doi.org/10.1155/2015/103570.

35. Wagner J. Incorporating acupressure into nursing practice. Am J Nurs 2015; 115(12):40–5.

36. Yen CH, Chien LC, Suen LKP. Application of auricular therapy for cancer-related pain in nursing care. J Pain Relief 2014;3(2). http://dx.doi.org/10.4172/2167-0846.1000139.

37. Chen H, Ning Z, Lam WL, et al. Types of control in acupuncture clinical trials might affect the conclusion of the trials: a review of acupuncture on pain management. J Acupunct Meridian Stud 2016;9(5):227–33.

38. Chen Y-W, Wang H-H. The effectiveness of acupressure on relieving pain: a systematic review. Pain Manag Nurs 2014;15(2):539–50.

39. Kober A, Scheck T, Greher M, et al. Prehospital anesthesia with acupressure at the Baihui and Hegu points in patients with radial fractures: a prospective, randomized, double-blind trial. Anesth Analg 2002;95(3):1328–32.

40. Johnson A, Kent P, Swanson B, et al. The use of acupuncture for pain management in pediatric patients. Altern Complement Ther 2015;21(6):255–60.

41. Park E, Oh H, Kim T. The effects of relaxation breathing on procedural pain and anxiety during burn care. Burns 2013;39(6):1101–6.

42. Zautra AJ, Fasman R, Davis MC, et al. The effects of slow breathing on affective responses to pain stimuli: an experimental study. Pain 2009;149:12–8.

43. Busch V, Magerl W, Kern U, et al. The effect of deep and slow breathing on pain perception, autonomic activity, and mood processing—an experimental study. Pain Med 2012;13:215–28.

44. Relaxation techniques for health. National Center for Complementary and Integrative Health. Available at: https://nccih.nih.gov/health/stress/relaxation.htm#hed3. Accessed April 1, 2016.

45. Complementary therapies. College of Nurses of Ontario. Available at: https://www.cno.org/globalassets/docs/prac/41021_comptherapies.pdf. Accessed March 24, 2017.

Dyspnea

Margaret L. Campbell, PhD, RN, FPCN

KEYWORDS

- Dyspnea • Respiratory distress • Critical care • Assessment • Treatment

KEY POINTS

- Dyspnea is highly prevalent in the intensive care unit, including in patients undergoing mechanical ventilation.
- Dyspnea is one of the most distressing symptoms experienced by critically ill patients; it can be likened to suffocation.
- Assessment may be hampered by the patient's inability to communicate or self-report secondary to intubation and/or cognitive impairment.
- Treating the underlying condition is the first step to relieving dyspnea.
- A number of evidence-based interventions may relieve the dyspnea sensation.

INTRODUCTION

Dyspnea is a subjective experience of breathing discomfort that consists of qualitatively distinct sensations that vary in intensity and can only be known through the patient's report.[1] Dyspnea is akin to suffocation and is one of the worst symptoms experienced by critically ill patients, including those who are mechanically ventilated.[2] When a patient cannot report dyspnea, as typifies many critically ill patients, the observed behaviors are characterized as respiratory distress.[3]

Expert guidelines are available to assist in the management of dyspnea,[1,4] but additional empirical evidence to support clinical care is needed, and wide variation persists in practice. The purpose of this paper is to address the following questions: (1) How prevalent, intense, and distressing is dyspnea experienced by critically ill patients? (2) How should dyspnea be assessed in the intensive care unit (ICU)? (3) What are current strategies for managing dyspnea during critical illness?

DYSPNEA MECHANISMS

The pathophysiologic basis for dyspnea occurs when there is a derangement in respiratory function. Normal respiration is a function of the complex integration of the respiratory control system consisting of voluntary, autonomic and emotional responses.

The author has nothing to disclose.
College of Nursing, Wayne State University, 5557 Cass Avenue, #344, Detroit, MI 48202, USA
E-mail address: m.campbell@wayne.edu

Crit Care Nurs Clin N Am 29 (2017) 461–470
http://dx.doi.org/10.1016/j.cnc.2017.08.006
0899-5885/17/© 2017 Elsevier Inc. All rights reserved.

Conscious controls (voluntary) from the cortex were identified in functional MRI studies of healthy human subjects during volitional breathing.[5–7] The autonomic responses are regulated in the brainstem and are basic and vital to the existence of the organism and will override conscious controls. Hence, telling a dyspneic patient to slow down their breathing is a futile exercise (**Fig. 1**).

Respiratory sensors consist of central (medulla, pons) and peripheral chemoreceptors (aortic and carotid bodies) and peripheral sensory receptors found in the chest wall, airways, and lungs. Alterations in respiratory function will produce blood gas imbalances (hypoxemia and hypercarbia) and changes in thoracic displacement. Peripheral afferents play only a minor role in respiratory control.

Stimulation of the respiratory center elicits an increased respiratory and cardiac response through activation of the parabrachial complex in the pons,[8] sympathetic nervous system, and activation of the adrenal medullary catecholamines (epinephrine and norepinephrine). Increased cardiac and pulmonary responses from central respiratory control and the sympathetic nervous system produces compensatory responses, including accelerations in heart and respiratory rates, increased lung volumes through recruitment of thoracic accessory muscles, changes in muscle tone, and increases in mean arterial pressure.[9] These cardiorespiratory responses are intended to restore respiratory homeostasis and preserve life.

The awareness of difficulty breathing, dyspnea, and the associated emotional responses of fear and anxiety are produced when there is pathology compromising normal respiratory functioning and is characterized by antecedent conditions, neurophysiologic, pulmonary, and emotional responses, and patient subjective experiences and behaviors.[10]

ANTECEDENT CONDITIONS AND MECHANISMS

A number of common pathologic conditions produce dyspnea (**Table 1**). The physiologic conditions shown in **Table 1** have 1 or more common mechanisms for producing uncomfortable breathing, including respiratory effort, blood gas imbalances, and afferent mismatch. A sense of respiratory effort is produced by conscious awareness of voluntary activation of the diaphragm, intercostals, and sternocleidomastoid muscles. Muscle receptors provide feedback about muscle force and tension, and information from these chest wall receptors produce the conscious awareness of respiratory effort. The respiratory muscles also activate autonomic central respiratory motor centers (ventromedial pons and medulla) that can contribute to the sense of effort.

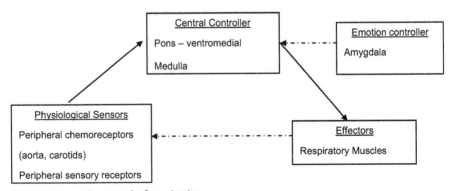

Fig. 1. Autonomic control of respiration.

Table 1
Conditions that produce dyspnea

Systems	Disorders
Pulmonary	Asthma
	Adult respiratory distress syndrome
	Chronic obstructive pulmonary disease
	Cystic fibrosis
	Interstitial lung disease
	Lung cancer, primary or metastatic
	Pleural effusion
	Pneumonia
	Pneumothorax
	Pulmonary arterial hypertension
	Pulmonary embolism
	Radiation pneumonitis
Cardiovascular	Heart failure
	Congenital heart anomalies
	Superior vena cava syndrome
Neuromuscular	Amyotrophic lateral sclerosis
	Muscular dystrophy
	Multiple sclerosis
	Myasthenia gravis
	Deconditioning
Miscellaneous	Hypervolemia
	Anemia

Sense of effort arises from awareness of the motor command generated during a breathing task. One theory proposes that, during voluntary activation of muscles, a corollary discharge is sent from the oligosynaptic corticospinal pathway to the pontomedullary respiratory centers at the same time that the efferent command is sent to the muscles, this corollary discharge is sensed as effort.[11] The sense of effort increases when the respiratory muscles are fatigued or deconditioned,[12] when there is an increased elastic or resistive load,[13] or when the level of ventilation is increased.[14]

Hypercapnia and hypoxemia have long been known to produce an involuntary motor response mediated in the brainstem to increase ventilation through increased rate and volume of breathing. Increased volume is achieved through activation of the accessory muscles (intercostals and sternocleidomastoid) via the ventromedial pons. This increased recruitment of accessory muscles produces the previously discussed increased sense of effort that correlates with dyspnea. Hypercapnia and hypoxemia also make independent contributions to the sensation of dyspnea.[14] Hypercarbia produced reports of dyspnea and fear when the partial pressure of carbon dioxide (Pco_2) increased by 5 to 10 mm Hg from the person's baseline level.[15,16] Severe hypercarbia (Pco_2 >80 mm Hg) produces a narcotic effect that will arguably inhibit emotions and, at very high levels suppresses, the brainstem respiratory center causing death.[17–19] Moosavi and colleagues[20] (2003) demonstrated that hypoxemia also has critical thresholds. Air hunger ratings increased sharply when levels of oxygen decreased to 50 mm Hg or less. Severe, persistent hypoxemia contributes to global brain ischemia and suppression of all brain functions until total brain death occurs.

In addition, a mismatch between afferent information (chemical and mechanical) and outgoing motor commands from the brainstem produces dyspnea. When subjects received an inspiratory flow less than that which they identified as most comfortable, they experienced dyspnea.[21] Other investigators demonstrated that healthy subjects are more comfortable when the mode of mechanical ventilation is such that the pattern is determined by the subject than when the pattern is imposed.[22] These studies suggest that a deviation from an expected pattern of ventilation will produce an increase in uncomfortable respiratory sensations.

Pathologic conditions that produce dyspnea do so by more than one mechanism. However, sense of effort is shared by most of the pathologic conditions, including asthma, chronic obstructive pulmonary disease (COPD), congestive heart failure, interstitial lung disease, and neuromuscular conditions.[14] Hypoxemia and hypercarbia are also common to all the pathologic conditions that produce dyspnea particularly during severe exacerbations and respiratory failure.

PREVALENCE, INTENSITY, AND DISTRESS IN THE INTENSIVE CARE UNIT

Studies conducted in various ICU settings confirm that dyspnea is among the most prevalent, intense, and distressing physical symptoms experienced by critically ill patients who can provide a symptom self-report. In a study of critically ill patients with cancer receiving ICU care, 34% of those who could self-report symptoms experienced moderate or severe dyspnea.[23] In another study of more than 400 interviews with 171 critically ill patients at high risk of dying revealed dyspnea in 44% of assessments.[2] Among those receiving mechanical ventilation, another investigator showed that almost one-half of patients experienced dyspnea.[24] The symptom experience of cognitively impaired patients, as typifies the critically ill and/or dying patient, is less well-understood.[25]

ASSESSMENT

The cornerstone of effective symptom control is systematic symptom assessment. Ideally, symptoms are reported and rated by patients themselves, using a tool that is sufficiently simple and brief to avoid burden while providing adequate information for clinical use. The Condensed Form of the Memorial Symptom Assessment Scale[26] and the Edmonton Symptom Assessment Scale[27] are tools of this kind that measure a diverse group of physical symptoms including dyspnea and psychological symptoms. In addition, a 10-item symptom scale incorporating 10 symptoms was validated in a large group of ICU patients.[2]

Brief, symptom-specific tools are also available to obtain self-reports of dyspnea. For patients who are unable to speak because of endotracheal intubation or other reasons, clinicians should provide opportunities to report through head shaking (yes/no) or pointing on a visual analog scale. Gift[28] found that a vertical visual analog scale was preferred by patients for reporting dyspnea.

When the patient is able to report but not verbalize symptom information, there may be a role for speech language pathologists to help augment the patient's ability to communicate and to assist communication through alternative approaches.[29] Simple strategies include alphabet and numbers boards, although more sophisticated modalities include electronic speech-generating devices or a touch screen requiring minimal physical pressure to activate message buttons.[29]

Although some patients may be unable to provide a dyspnea self-report, we cannot assume that they are unable to experience respiratory distress. Although other symptom information is less accurate than the patient's own report, the symptom intensity and/or distress of critically ill patients who cannot provide self-reports must still be addressed. Two main approaches have been used for this purpose: (1) behavioral assessment and (2) proxy assessment.

Behavioral Symptom Assessment

The Respiratory Distress Observation Scale (RDOS) is the only known behavioral scale for assessment of respiratory distress when a patient cannot report dyspnea (**Table 2**). RDOS is an ordinal scale with 8 observer-rated parameters: heart rate, respiratory rate, accessory muscle use, paradoxical breathing pattern, restlessness, grunting at end-expiration, nasal flaring, and a fearful facial display. Each parameter is scored from 0 to 2 points and the points are summed. Scale scores range from 0 signifying no distress to 16 signifying the most severe distress Behavior variables that comprise the RDOS were identified from videotaping mechanically ventilated patients undergoing a failed ventilator weaning trial and experiencing naturally occurring dyspnea.[30] Construct validity was established through correlation with hypoxemia[31,32] and use of oxygen.[32] The internal consistency across studies has ranged from an α of 0.64 to 0.86.[31,32] Interrater reliability was perfect between data collectors (r = 1.0). Convergent validity was established through comparison with dyspnea self-report on a visual analog scale.[31] Discriminant validity was established with comparisons of RDOS from COPD patients with dyspnea to patients with acute pain and healthy volunteers.[31] Distress intensity cutpoints were established: 0 to 2 (no distress), 3 (mild distress), 4 to 6 (signifies moderate distress), and 7 or more (severe distress).[33,34]

Proxy Symptom Assessment

The use of symptom reports from surrogates, such as family members, or clinicians themselves, in various patient populations remains controversial. In some studies, patients rank their symptoms higher than proxy reporters,[35] whereas in other reports the opposite is true.[36,37]

Table 2
Respiratory Distress Observation Scale

Variable	0 Points	1 Point	2 Points	Total
Heart rate per minute	<90 beats	90–109 beats	≥110 beats	
Respiratory rate per minute	≤18 breaths	19–30 breaths	>30 breaths	
Restlessness: nonpurposeful movements	None	Occasional, slight movements	Frequent movements	
Accessory muscle use: rise in clavicle during inspiration	None	Slight rise	Pronounced rise	
Paradoxical breathing pattern: abdomen moves in on inspiration	None		Present	
Grunting at end-expiration: guttural sound	None		Present	
Nasal flaring: involuntary movement of nares	None		Present	
Look of fear	None		Eyes wide open, facial muscles tense, brow furrowed, mouth open	
Total				

WHAT ARE CURRENT STRATEGIES FOR MANAGING DYSPNEA DURING CRITICAL ILLNESS?

The first line is to treat dyspnea by optimizing the management of the underlying etiologic condition such as with inotropes and diuretics for heart failure exacerbations, bronchodilators for COPD, thoracentesis, or antibiotics to name a few. Mechanical ventilation, either invasive or noninvasive, is the most reliable means of reducing dyspnea from respiratory failure, although not without the well-understood burdens to the patient. Some patients will not want to undergo mechanical ventilation and the treatment of dyspnea must rely on other interventions, such as those directed at relieving the sensation of dyspnea and the associated emotional response; these may be effective singly or in combination (**Table 3**).

Optimal positioning is patient specific. For example, dyspnea in COPD is effectively reduced by upright positioning with arms elevated on pillows or a bedside table.[38,39] In unilateral lung disease the patient may find a side-lying position optimal with the "good" lung up or down to increase perfusion and/or ventilation. Using the patient as his or her own control and measuring dyspnea or respiratory distress in various positions permits identification of the optimal position. Patient activity, whether active or passive, increases oxygen consumption and may lead to dyspnea. Nurses coordinate all patient care and are integral to ensuring staggering of activity to minimize or prevent dyspnea.

Oxygen is useful to reduce dyspnea caused by hypoxemia. However, no benefit from oxygen compared with medical air was found in a multinational study of patients with advanced lung disease who were not hypoxemic.[40] Furthermore, patients who were near death and at risk for dyspnea remained comfortable without oxygen.[41] A fan directed at the dyspneic patients face may provide relief,[42] although use in the ICU may be limited by bioengineering restrictions.

Opioids, most commonly immediate release oral morphine or intravenous fentanyl, are the mainstay of pharmacologic management of dyspnea that is refractory to disease-modifying treatment, and its effectiveness has been demonstrated in clinical trials.[43] Effectiveness has not been established for other opioids such as hydromorphone or hydrocodone, or other routes such as transdermal or intravenous. The doses of opioids for acute dyspnea exacerbations are less well-known than those used to treat acute pain; "low and slow" titration of an immediate release form given intravenously, and repeated every 15 minutes should be provided until the patient reports or displays relief. Around the clock dosing may be best if the patient has dyspnea continuously or at rest, but with as-needed dosing for episodic dyspnea.[44] The constipating effect of opioids never abates and all patients receiving opioids must be on a bowel regimen such as senna.

The effectiveness of benzodiazepines as a primary treatment for dyspnea has not been established.[45] The addition of a benzodiazepine as an adjunct to the opioid regimen has been successful in patients with advanced COPD.[46,47] Benzodiazepines are effective for treating anxiety, which is often a parallel symptom with dyspnea. As with opioids, these agents should be titrated to effect.

Nebulized furosemide has shown equivocal results in case reports of reducing dyspnea in advanced disease.[48–51] The putative advantage of furosemide over opioids is the lack of serious side effects, such as hypotension and fears about respiratory depression; however, effectiveness has not been established.

Treating patients' dyspnea in the presence of physiologic instability is an ongoing concern for ICU clinicians. Fears of hypotension, respiratory depression, sedation, and addiction can lead to physician reluctance to prescribe an opioid and to nurse

Table 3
Dyspnea interventions, mode of action, and rationale

Intervention	Dose	Mode of Action	Rationale	Outcome
Optimal positioning, usually upright with arms elevated and supported[38,39]	Whenever patient reports dyspnea or displays respiratory distress	Increased pulmonary volume capacity	Increases air exchange, which may improve oxygenation and carbon dioxide clearance, and reduce inspiratory effort	Reduced dyspnea or respiratory distress
Balance rest with activity Stagger nursing care	Guided by dyspnea/ respiratory distress	Decreases excessive oxygen consumption	Prevents hypoxemia	Reduced dyspnea/respiratory distress
Oxygen as indicated by goals of therapy; not useful in normoxemia or when the patient is near death and in no distress[40,41,55]	Variable, guided by goals of therapy and patient characteristics	Improves the partial pressure of oxygen; reduces lactic acidemia	Treats hypoxemia	Patient report or display of reduced respiratory distress. Oxygen saturation is not a measure of dyspnea/ respiratory distress
Cold cloth on face[56]	As needed	Trigeminal nerve stimulation; action on dyspnea unknown	Anecdotal reports of patient relief; inexpensive; easy to perform	Reduced dyspnea/respiratory distress
Morphine or fentanyl[43]	Low doses titrated to the patient's report of dyspnea or display of dyspnea behaviors is effective; oral or parenteral; no evidence to support inhaled; no evidence on dosing regimens	Uncertain direct effect; reduced brainstem sensitivity to oxygen and carbon dioxide[1]; altered central nervous perception[44]	Strong evidence-base supports effectiveness	Reduced dyspnea/respiratory distress
Benzodiazepines, such as lorazepam or midazolam[46]	Low doses titrated to the patient's report of anxiety or display of anxiety behaviors; no evidence for benzodiazepine regimens	Anxiolysis	Fear or anxiety often accompanies dyspnea.	Reduced anxiety

administration of suboptimal doses.[52] Clinician fears about respiratory depression are in contradiction to the evidence; no patients in studies of opioid use for dyspnea experienced respiratory depression.[43,53,54] Clinicians are advised to consider patient comfort as a priority and, in so doing, call on the use of interdisciplinary communication, assessment, decision making, and drug titration skills to provide relief for all patients.

SUMMARY

Alleviation of respiratory distress is a core element of care in the ICU. An important goal for ICU care improvement is to not only promote patient comfort, but to support other favorable outcomes of intensive care that are associated with dyspnea control. Selection of dyspnea assessment methods to meet the specific communication abilities of the patient is necessary to gain as much knowledge of what the patient is experiencing as possible. Selection of dyspnea management techniques appropriate to the source, or anticipated source, of the symptom, the condition of the patient, and the goals of care requires the concerted efforts of a dedicated team of multidisciplinary health care professionals.

REFERENCES

1. Parshall MB, Schwartzstein RM, Adams L, et al. An official American Thoracic Society statement: update on the mechanisms, assessment, and management of dyspnea. Am J Respir Crit Care Med 2012;185(4):435–52.
2. Puntillo KA, Arai S, Cohen NH, et al. Symptoms experienced by intensive care unit patients at high risk of dying. Crit Care Med 2010;38(11):2155–60.
3. Campbell ML. Terminal dyspnea and respiratory distress. Crit Care Clin 2004; 20(3):403–17.
4. Mahler DA, Selecky PA, Harrod CG. Management of dyspnea in patients with advanced lung or heart disease: practical guidance from the American college of chest physicians consensus statement. Pol Arch Med Wewn 2010;120(5): 160–6.
5. Evans KC, Shea SA, Saykin AJ. Functional MRI localisation of central nervous system regions associated with volitional inspiration in humans. J Physiol 1999; 520:383–92.
6. McKay LC, Evans KC, Frackowiak RS, et al. Neural correlates of voluntary breathing in humans. J Appl Physiol 2003;95:1170–8.
7. Horn EM, Waldrop TG. Suprapontine control of respiration. Respir Physiol 1998; 114:201–11.
8. Chamberlin NL, Saper CB. A brainstem network mediating apneic reflexes in the rat. J Neurosci 1998;18:6048–56.
9. West JB. Respiratory physiology: the essentials. Philadelphia: Lippincott, Williams and Wilkins; 1999.
10. Burki NK, Tobin MJ, Guz A, et al. Dyspnea: mechanisms, evaluation and treatment. Am Rev Respir Dis 1988;138(4):1040–1.
11. McCloskey DI. Corollary discharges: motor commands and perception. In: Brookhart JM, Mountcastle VB, editors. The nervous system: handbook of physiology. Bethesda (MD): American Physiological Society; 1981. p. 1415–47.
12. Gandevia SC, Killian KJ, Campbell EJM. The effect of respiratory muscle fatigue on respiratory sensations. Clin Sci 1981;60:463–6.
13. Redline S, Gottfried SB, Altose MD. Effect of changes in inspiratory muscle strength on the sensation of respiratory force. J Appl Physiol 1991;70:240–5.

14. Manning HL, Schwartzstein RM. Mechanisms of dyspnea. In: Mahler DA, editor. Dyspnea. New York: Marcel Decker, Inc; 1998. p. 63–95.
15. Banzett RB, Lansing RW, Reid MB, et al. 'Air hunger' arising from increased pCO_2 in mechanically ventilated quadriplegics. Respir Physiol 1989;76:53–68.
16. Banzett RB, Lansing RW, Evans KC, et al. Stimulus-response characteristics of CO_2-induced air hunger in normal subjects. Respir Physiol 1996;103:19–31.
17. Taxen DV. Permissive hypercapnea. In: Tobin MJ, editor. Principles and practices of mechanical ventilation. New York: McGraw-Hill Book Co; 1994.
18. Reid KH, Patenaude B, Guo SZ, et al. Carbon dioxide narcosis-induced apnea in a rat model of cardiac arrest and resuscitation. Resuscitation 1998;38:185–91.
19. Dean JB, Mulkey DK, Garcia AJ 3rd, et al. Neuronal sensitivity to hyperoxia, hypercapnia, and inert gases at hyperbaric pressures. J Appl Physiol 2003;95: 883–909.
20. Moosavi SH, Golestanian E, Binks AP, et al. Hypoxic and hypercapnic drives to breathe generate equivalent levels of air hunger in humans. J Appl Physiol 2003;94:141–54.
21. Manning HL, Molinary E, Leiter JC. Effect of inspiratory flow on respiratory sensation and pattern of breathing. Am J Respir Crit Care Med 1995;151:751–7.
22. Russell WC, Greer JR. The comfort of breathing: a study with volunteers assessing the influence of various modes of assisted ventilation. Crit Care Med 2000; 28(11):3645–8.
23. Nelson JE, Meier DE, Oei EJ, et al. Self-reported symptom experience of critically ill cancer patients receiving intensive care. Crit Care Med 2001;29(2):277–82.
24. Schmidt M, Demoule A, Polito A, et al. Dyspnea in mechanically ventilated critically ill patients. Crit Care Med 2011;39(9):2059–65.
25. Campbell ML. Dyspnea prevalence, trajectories, and measurement in critical care and at life's end. Curr Opin Support Palliat Care 2012;6(2):168–71.
26. Chang VT, Hwang SS, Thaler HT, et al. Memorial symptom assessment scale. Expert Rev Pharmacoecon Outcomes Res 2004;4(2):171–8.
27. Bruera E, Kuehn N, Miller MJ, et al. The Edmonton Symptom Assessment System (ESAS): a simple method for the assessment of palliative care patients. J Palliat Care 1991;7(2):6–9.
28. Gift A. Validation of a vertical visual analogue scale as a measure of clinical dyspnea. Rehabil Nurs 1989;14:323–5.
29. Radtke JV, Baumann BM, Garrett KL, et al. Listening to the voiceless patient: case reports in assisted communication in the intensive care unit. J Palliat Med 2011; 14(6):791–5.
30. Campbell ML. Fear and pulmonary stress behaviors to an asphyxial threat across cognitive states. Res Nurs Health 2007;30(6):572–83.
31. Campbell ML. Psychometric testing of a respiratory distress observation scale. J Palliat Med 2008;11(1):44–50.
32. Campbell ML, Templin T, Walch J. A respiratory distress observation scale for patients unable to self-report dyspnea. J Palliat Med 2010;13(3):285–90.
33. Campbell ML, Templin TN. Intensity cut-points for the respiratory distress observation scale. Palliat Med 2015;29(5):436–42.
34. Campbell ML, Templin TN, Kero KK. Mild, moderate and severe cut-points for the respiratory distress observation scale: a receiver operating characteristic curve analysis. J Pain Symptom Manage 2016;51(2):342–3.
35. Haugdahl HS, Storli SL, Meland B, et al. Underestimation of patient breathlessness by nurses and physicians during a spontaneous breathing trial. Am J Respir Crit Care Med 2015;192(12):1440–8.

36. Puntillo KA, Neuhaus J, Arai S, et al. Challenge of assessing symptoms in seriously ill intensive care unit patients: can proxy reporters help? Crit Care Med 2012;40(10):2760–7.
37. Kutner JS, Bryant LL, Beaty BL, et al. Symptom distress and quality-of-life assessment at the end of life: the role of proxy response. J Pain Symptom Manage 2006;32(4):300–10.
38. Barach AL. Chronic obstructive lung disease: postural relief of dyspnea. Arch Phys Med Rehabil 1974;55:494–504.
39. Sharp JT, Drutz WS, Moisan T, et al. Postural relief of dyspnea in severe chronic obstructive lung disease. Am Rev Respir Dis 1980;122:201–11.
40. Abernethy AP, McDonald CF, Frith PA, et al. Effect of palliative oxygen versus room air in relief of breathlessness in patients with refractory dyspnoea: a double-blind, randomised controlled trial. Lancet 2010;376(9743):784–93.
41. Campbell ML, Yarandi H, Dove-Medows E. Oxygen is nonbeneficial for most patients who are near death. J Pain Symptom Manage 2013;45(3):517–23.
42. Bausewein C, Booth S, Gysels M, et al. Effectiveness of a hand-held fan for breathlessness: a randomised phase II trial. BMC Palliat Care 2010;9:22.
43. Jennings AL, Davies AN, Higgins JP, et al. A systematic review of the use of opioids in the management of dyspnoea. Thorax 2002;57(11):939–44.
44. Rocker G, Horton R, Currow D, et al. Palliation of dyspnoea in advanced COPD: revisiting a role for opioids. Thorax 2009;64(10):910–5.
45. Simon ST, Higginson IJ, Booth S, et al. Benzodiazepines for the relief of breathlessness in advanced malignant and non-malignant diseases in adults. Cochrane Database Syst Rev 2010;(1):CD007354.
46. Navigante AH, Cerchietti LC, Castro MA, et al. Midazolam as adjunct therapy to morphine in the alleviation of severe dyspnea perception in patients with advanced cancer. J Pain Symptom Manage 2006;31(1):38–47.
47. Sironi O, Sbanotto A, Banfi MG, et al. Midazolam as adjunct therapy to morphine to relieve dyspnea? J Pain Symptom Manage 2007;33(3):233–4 [author reply: 234–6].
48. Kohara H, Ueoka H, Aoe K, et al. Effect of nebulized furosemide in terminally ill cancer patients with dyspnea. J Pain Symptom Manage 2003;26(4):962–7.
49. Stone P, Rix, Kurowska A, et al. Re: nebulized furosemide for dyspnea in terminal cancer patients. J Pain Symptom Manage 2002;24(3):274–5 [author reply: 275–6].
50. Shimoyama N, Shimoyama M. Nebulized furosemide as a novel treatment for dyspnea in terminal cancer patients. J Pain Symptom Manage 2002;23(1):73–6.
51. Wilcock A, Walton A, Manderson C, et al. Randomised, placebo controlled trial of nebulised furosemide for breathlessness in patients with cancer. Thorax 2008; 63(10):872–5.
52. Pasero C, Puntillo K, Li D, et al. Structured approaches to pain management in the ICU. Chest 2009;135(6):1665–72.
53. Banzett RB, Adams L, O'Donnell CR, et al. Using laboratory models to test treatment: morphine reduces dyspnea and hypercapnic ventilatory response. Am J Respir Crit Care Med 2011;184(8):920–7.
54. Currow DC, McDonald C, Oaten S, et al. Once-daily opioids for chronic dyspnea: a dose increment and pharmacovigilance study. J Pain Symptom Manage 2011; 42(3):388–99.
55. Mahler DA, Selecky PA, Harrod CG, et al. American College of Chest Physicians consensus statement on the management of dyspnea in patients with advanced lung or heart disease. Chest 2010;137(3):674–91.
56. Schwartzstein RM, Lahive K, Pope A, et al. Cold facial stimulation reduces breathlessness induced in normal subjects. Am Rev Respir Dis 1987;136:58–61.

Pain Management in Obstetrics

Jennifer G. Hensley, EdD, CNM, WHNP, LCCE[a,*], Michelle R. Collins, PhD, CNM[b],
Claire L. Leezer, MSN, CNM[b]

KEYWORDS

- Pain in labor • Suffering in labor • Pharmacologic pain management in labor
- Nonpharmacologic pain management in labor

KEY POINTS

- The pain of labor pain is a complex, multidimensional phenomenon that is experienced with great individual variation between women.
- There are a multitude of options that may be safely used to alleviate pain in labor, both pharmacologic and nonpharmacologic.
- When women desire alleviation of labor pain, clinicians need to carefully consider the hormonal and physiologic changes of pregnancy, the modality of pain relief and its efficacy, as well as risks, benefits, and contraindications.

INTRODUCTION: NATURE OF PAIN DURING LABOR

"Unlike other acute and chronic pain experiences, labor pain is not associated with pathology but with the most basic and fundamental of life's experiences—the bringing forth of new life."[1] Pain, as it relates to any other organic process—disease, injury, dying—may well equate to suffering. Suffering, in contrast, is a complex psychological response mediated by a number of factors, not the least of which are fear and anxiety.

Pain and suffering are not equal when applied to childbirth. Unlike the physiologic pain associated with injury or a disease process, the pain involved in childbirth is described as "pain with a purpose." Although women experience a varying degree of physiologic pain in childbirth, to assume that all women suffer negates the innumerable variables that contribute to suffering that include prior experience, social support, circumstances of labor and birth, and even whether or not the pregnancy was desired.

Disclosure Statement: No authors have anything to disclosure.
[a] School of Nursing, University of Texas Austin, 1710 Red River Street, Austin, TX 78701, USA;
[b] Nurse-Midwifery Program, University Nurse-Midwifery Practice, Vanderbilt University School of Nursing, 461 – 21st Street South, Nashville, TN 37421, USA
* Corresponding author.
E-mail address: JHensley@pcisys.net

Crit Care Nurs Clin N Am 29 (2017) 471–485
http://dx.doi.org/10.1016/j.cnc.2017.08.007
0899-5885/17/© 2017 Elsevier Inc. All rights reserved.

ccnursing.theclinics.com

Labor pain is a complex, multidimensional phenomenon that is experienced with great individual variation, but certain physiologic aspects are universal. During the first stage of labor, stretching and distention of the lower uterine segment, as well as dilation of the cervix, stimulate mechanoreceptors, which serve to transmit painful impulses. These impulses traverse visceral sympathetic nerves at T10 through L1 along the spinal cord.[2] During the second stage, the pain of perineal stretching stimulates somatic nerves, which transmit impulses through the pudendal and sacral nerves that enter the spinal cord at S2 through S4.[2] Although a woman's experience of labor pain, and her response to it, are influenced by emotional, motivational, cognitive, social, and cultural factors, perception of pain and the ability to cope with it are modified by fear and anxiety.[2] Unmitigated pain during childbirth can have adverse implications for maternal and fetal health. Increased activity of the sympathetic nervous system results in a surge of catecholamines.[2,3] Hyperventilation and an increased metabolic rate result in greater oxygen consumption and can lead to hypocarbia and hypoxemia. Increased maternal blood pressure can develop in response to greater cardiac output and vascular resistance.[2,3] The interplay of these cardiopulmonary alterations can ultimately lead to an uncoordinated uterine contraction pattern with decreased uteroplacental perfusion that results in fetal hypoxemia and fetal acidosis.[2,3] To help alleviate pain and suffering during childbirth, obstetric analgesia and anesthesia and nonpharmacologic modalities will be discussed.

HISTORY OF PAIN MANAGEMENT IN OBSTETRICS

In 1846, Boston dentist William Morton demonstrated the use of ether as an anesthetic. Shortly thereafter, Scottish obstetrician and midwifery professor James Simpson, administered ether inhalation to a woman with a contracted pelvis to rotate and extract the fetus for a vaginal delivery.[4] He also demonstrated the separate use of nitrous oxide (N_2O) and chloroform as alternative agents for labor pain.[4] Chloroform had multiple adverse effects and was, in fact, responsible for a number of deaths. Nonetheless, despite overarching disapproval from the medical profession, obstetric anesthesia was accepted into practice owing to public pressure.[5] By 1900, approximately 50% of all physician-attended births involved the use of either ether or chloroform.[6]

In 1902, Austrian physician Richard von Steinbuchel was the first to introduce injectable scopolamine hydrobromide and morphine sulfate, which resulted in an amnesic–analgesic state during labor.[7,8] In 1915, the National Twilight Sleep Association was established and was credited with the adoption of "twilight sleep" that became the standard for obstetric anesthesia in the United States.[9] Concerns over the safety of twilight sleep did not arise until one of its most avid supporters, Francis X. Carmody, died in childbirth, although her death was not related to twilight sleep.[7] Nonetheless, continued widespread use led to the misuse of morphine and subsequent asphyxiation of babies.[8] In 1900, Swiss obstetrician Oscar Kreis introduced regional anesthesia when he injected cocaine into the spine of 6 laboring women. Despite high rates of vomiting and headaches, regional anesthesia was well-received. Unfortunately, high rates of mortality were noted owing, in large part, to inexperienced attendants and inadequate monitoring.[10] Between 1900 and 1930, newer and safer options for obstetric anesthesia and analgesia were developed, which included the lumbar epidural, caudal, paravertebral, parasacral, pudendal, and newer inhalation and intravenous agents.[7] In 1931, Romanian Eugen Aburel developed the continuous lumbar epidural block.[11] This was a breakthrough, because this form of pain management enabled women to be fully conscious during birth without risk of maternal toxicity, adverse effects on the fetus, or obstruction of labor. From the 1940s forward, advances in regional anesthesia continued such that, by 1970, epidural use became (and remains) a standard of practice for management of pain in labor.[10]

Concerns related to obstetric analgesia and anesthesia birthed the "natural childbirth" movement. In 1913, British obstetrician Grantly Dick-Read, developed a technique that involved the education of women on the process of childbirth with the requirement they actively participate in the birth process.[6] Specific breathing patterns and muscle relaxation during simulated contractions "reprogrammed" the woman's anticipation of, and response to, the pain of childbirth. Use of these psychoprophylactic techniques significantly decreased fear and anxiety. Later, the Lamaze method gained worldwide popularity and initiated the broader psychoprophylaxis movement[6] with the development of other nonpharmacologic modalities that include the Bradley Method, the Alexander Technique, and hypnobirthing, all of which can be used alone or in combination with pharmacologic methods (**Table 1**).

PHYSIOLOGIC CHANGES DURING PREGNANCY

Pregnancy is a time of dynamic anatomic and physiologic change.[2] Blood volume can double, leading to changes in vital signs and laboratory results. The enlarging, gravid uterus displaces abdominal and thoracic organs and puts pressure on the inferior vena cava and aorta, which can obstruct blood flow from and to the heart.[2] A review of these physiologic changes in pregnancy is offered in **Table 2**.

TYPES OF PAIN MANAGEMENT
Injectables

Management of labor pain helps to mitigate fear and anxiety and the subsequent release of catecholamines that can have adverse maternal and fetal consequences, as mentioned earlier. Injectable analgesics (intravenous, intramuscular, and subcutaneous) with opioid and opioid agonist–antagonist properties provide relief of pain (**Table 3**). These agents typically have a short half-life that requires frequent administration, making the use of a patient-controlled analgesia pump the preferred method. Injectable analgesics provide the woman with immediate pain relief, and use of a patient-controlled analgesia pump offers many women a sense of control. A concern with these agents is maternal and fetal/newborn sedation and respiratory depression, especially with meperidine (Demerol) and its metabolite normeperidine. Of all the opioids, fentanyl has gained popularity owing to its short half-life that results in fewer side effects. The use of intravenous promethazine or intramuscular hydroxyzine can potentiate the opioid analgesic and control for the side effects of nausea and vomiting.[37]

Inhalable Analgesic

Nitrous oxide (N_2O), and other inhalational agents like isoflurane and sevoflurane, have been used in obstetrics since 1846. Although widely used in Europe, N_2O experienced a decline in use in the United States once neuraxial anesthesia gained popularity. Today, N_2O is delivered via mask or mouthpiece, at a 50/50 concentration of nitrous oxide to oxygen, through an apparatus that is controlled completely by the laboring woman, adding an element of attraction for many women.

Women who are not candidates for neuraxial anesthesia, or who do not desire placement of a regional anesthetic, may desire and be candidates for N_2O use. Contraindications to N_2O use include acute drug or alcohol intoxication, impaired consciousness, recent history of trauma, pneumothorax, increased intracranial or intraocular pressure, bowel obstruction, middle ear surgery, emphysema, pulmonary

Table 1
Nonpharmacologic methods of pain management during childbirth

Method	Efficacy/Benefits	Contraindications	Risks
Psychoprophylaxis; prepares women to manage labor pain via use of breathing exercises and relaxation techniques.	Markedly decreased pain accompanied by greater degree of pain control and higher levels of satisfaction.[12]	None.	None.
Hydrotherapy: encompasses any use of therapeutic water during labor, whether complete immersion in a tub, or use of a shower.	Documented decreases in both duration of labor and pain intensity scores.[13–15] An integrative review noted a high degree of maternal satisfaction with pain relief and birth experience.[16] A Cochrane Systematic review noted a decrease in the use of neuraxial anesthesia, a mean reduction of 32 min in the first stage of labor and no increase in adverse effects or outcomes to either the mother or fetus when immersion was used.[18]	Labor before 37 wk of gestation, blood or skin infection, fever 100.4°F, abnormal vaginal bleeding, category II–III fetal heart rate tracing, suspected macrosomia with history of shoulder dystocia, malpresentation, or multiple gestation.[17] Prior cesarean birth is not an absolute contraindication.	None.
Acupressure/acupuncture	Mixed reviews as to efficacy for relieving pain in childbirth. Studies have noted usefulness in treating labor pain,[19–21] lower rates of neuraxial anesthesia,[22] and lower labor pain scores.[23] Overall, viable nonpharmacologic methods for pain relief in childbirth.	No contraindications specific to pregnancy that are not generalized for all. Some acupressure/acupuncture points should be avoided in preterm pregnancy. Some women may be averse to therapy involving needles.	Nausea and/or vomiting, altered taste, fatigue, treatment discomfort, and uterine contractions.[24]

Aromatherapy	The scents of lavender and bitter orange have proven to provide pain relief in childbirth.[25–27] Beyond simply an analgesic effect, the use of citrus aurantium and geranium oils have been shown efficacy in decreasing anxiety during childbirth.[28,29]	With the heightened olfactory sensitivity of pregnancy, some women may be averse to the strong scents. Skin contact with essential oils may result in irritation.	There is no evidence that addition of essential oils to water for labor or birth is safe for exposed neonates.
Music therapy	Markedly lower pain perception scores among women listening to music.[30–32] Similar to aromatherapy, music has a strong anxiolytic effect, thereby decreasing pain as a byproduct of anxiolysis.	None.	No documented adverse effect on either fetuses or neonates.
Meditation, mindfulness, and self-hypnosis: harnesses/focuses women's minds to claim power over physiologic labor pain, and accompanying anxiety and fear. Assists women to place "mind over matter" in relating to pain of labor and birth.	These require forethought and practice to be of greatest usefulness during childbirth. There is demonstrated efficacy noted in numerous studies.[33] A Cochrane review noted that women practicing self-hypnosis used less pharmacologic pain relief or analgesia, but not less regional anesthesia than control groups.	There are no contraindications. Altering states of consciousness have been deemed to directly conflict with basic Christian tenets and some women may object to these therapies, citing religious objection.	None.

Data from Refs.[12–33]

Table 2
Physiologic changes during pregnancy with changes in laboratory values

	Physiologic Adaptation	First Trimester (LMP to 12–3/7 wk)	Second Trimester (13–27–6/7 wk)	Third Trimester (28–40+ wk and birth)	Postpartum (Placenta to 42 d)	Comments
Plasma volume	Increase by 45%; greater increase in multifetal pregnancy	Increase begins 6–8 wk of gestation		Maximum volume at 32 wk		Nitric oxide vasodilation; stimulation of the renin–angiotensin–aldosterone system
RBC mass	Increase by 20%–30%			Increase by 250–450 mL		Increase in response to plasma volume
Hematocrit	Decrease	No change	Hemodilutional anemia (physiologic)	Peak hemodilutional anemia		Hemodilution owing to decrease in blood viscosity
Iron needs	Total requirement 1000 mg required for pregnancy					RBC mass expansion from increase in plasma volume and fetal iron needs in third trimester
Ventricular mass	Increase parallel to increase plasma volume	Increase		Maximal at 30 wk		Left ventricular torsion may protect against impaired diastolic function despite increase in preload
End-diastolic volume	Increase		Increase	Increase		
Cardiac output	Increase by 30%–50%	Increase seen by 8 wk of gestation				Increased owing plasma volume, ventricular mass, and end-diastolic volume

Renal blood flow	Increase by 50%		BUN and creatinine below nonpregnancy values
Uterine blood flow	Increase from 2% to 17% total cardiac output		
Serum albumin	Decrease by 12%–18%	Nadir at 24 wk	Susceptible to pulmonary edema
B-type natriuretic peptide	Increase 200%		
Systemic vascular resistance	Decrease by 30%	Nadir at 24 wk; Increase to prepregnancy baseline	Decrease paralleled by increase in plasma volume; reduced preload and afterload; vasodilation from progesterone and low-resistance placental bed
Tidal volume and minute ventilation	Increase by 40%		
Complete metabolic panel	Increase in CO_2; decrease in BUN, creatinine		Compensatory respiratory alkalosis; increased renal blood flow
Fasting and postprandial blood glucose	Decrease		

Abbreviations: BUN, blood urea nitrogen; LMP, last menstrual period; RBC, red blood cells.
Data from Refs.[2,34–37]

Table 3
Injectable analgesics

Drug	Class	Dose	Onset	Duration	Comments
Fentanyl	Opioid	25–50 µg IV PCA • Loading dose 50–100 µg IV • Bolus 10–25 µg IV • Lockout 5–12 min	1–3 min IV 1–3 min	30–60 min IV 30–60 min	Short-acting, potent respiratory depressant; best used by patient controlled anesthesia pump
Meperidine (Demerol)	Opioid	25–50 mg IV	5 min IV	2–3 h	Nausea and vomiting; active metabolite: normeperidine, a potent respiratory depressant; risk: neonatal respiratory depression most likely if birth between 1 and 4 h after administration
Morphine	Opioid	2–5 mg IV	3–5 min IV		Risk: neonatal respiratory depression
Nalbuphine (Nubain)	Mixed opioid agonist/antagonist	10 mg IV 10 mg IM	2–3 min IV 10–15 min IM	3–6 h	Less nausea and vomiting than with meperidine
Butorphanol (Stadol)	Mixed opioid agonist/antagonist	1–2 mg IV or IM	5–10 min IV 10–15 min IM 5–20 min IM	3–4 h	Maternal sedation similar to meperidine and phenothiazine; dysphoria
Promethazine (Phenergan)	Phenothiazine	25–75 mg IV/IM	10–20 min	3–4 h	Commonly used with opioids to mitigate nausea and vomiting; may produce hypotension
Hydroxyzine (Vistaril)	Antihistamine	25–50 mg IM only (in oil base)	30 min	4 h	Commonly used with opioids to mitigate nausea and vomiting

Abbreviations: IM, intramuscularly; IV, intravenously; PCA, patient-controlled analgesia.
Data from Refs.[37]

hypertension, and inability to hold mask over face. A documented vitamin B_{12} deficiency, such as is the case with certain malabsorptive conditions, is also a contraindication.[38-40] Side effects cause more discomfort than harm and include nausea and vomiting for approximately 10% of users. Fatigue after several hours of N_2O use has been noted, although it is unclear whether this fatigue is actually related to N_2O or to the physical work of labor. No adverse effects on fetuses have been noted.[41]

Neuraxial Anesthesia

Neuraxial anesthesia is currently the most common type of pain management used in obstetrics and includes the epidural block, spinal block, and combined spinal–epidural (CSE) block. According to the National Vital Statistics Report (2011), 61% of women who had a singleton birth in 2008 received spinal or epidural anesthesia.[42] For an epidural block, solutions of local anesthetic, opioids, or both, are administered, either by intermittent or continuous infusion, via a catheter passed through the ligamentum flavum into the lumbar epidural space.[43] For a CSE, a smaller gauge spinal needle is directed through the epidural needle, puncturing the dura and injecting a single bolus dose of an opioid, or a combination opioid and local anesthetic, into the subarachnoid space.[43] The relatively few contraindications to neuraxial anesthesia include maternal refusal or inability to cooperate during placement, coagulopathy and thrombocytopenia, skin or soft tissue infection at the site of needle placement, inadequate staffing or facilities, lack of immediately available resuscitative drugs or equipment, increased intracranial pressure (ICP) secondary to a mass, or uncorrected maternal hypovolemia (hemorrhage).[44]

The American College of Obstetricians and Gynecologists purports that, in the absence of a medical contraindication, a woman's desire for pain management is the only medical indication needed to provide neuraxial anesthesia.[45] This dense anesthetic technique can serve to modulate the pain response and subsequent release of catecholamines, thereby benefitting a woman who has a medical complication such as mitral stenosis, spinal cord injury, intracranial neurovascular disease, asthma, or preeclampsia.[46]

Side effects

Side effects of neuraxial anesthesia include hypotension, pruritus, nausea and vomiting, fever, shivering, and delayed gastric emptying.[46] Serious complications related to anesthesia in the obstetric population are rare, but include epidural abscess, epidural hematoma, transient or persistent neurologic injury, high neuraxial block necessitating endotracheal intubation, serious neurologic injury, postdural puncture headache, and fetal heart rate abnormalities.

Complications of neuraxial anesthesia

An epidural abscess occurs between the dura mater and the vertebral periosteum, most commonly in the lumbar spine region, with Staphylococcus aureus as the causative organism in 63.6% of cases.[47] Infection can arise from a break in aseptic technique during catheter placement, ascending infection from normal skin flora, contamination from local anesthetic syringes, or a preexisting infection.[48] The most common risk factors include diabetes mellitus and a history of intravenous drug abuse.[49] Symptoms may begin a few hours after administration or may not be present for a few weeks. The classic presentation includes site-specific pain, fever, and extremity weakness.[49] Other early symptoms include backache, headache, erythema, and tenderness at the site of insertion with progression to stiff neck, photophobia, radiating pain, loss of motor function, and confusion.[50]

Although the risk of epidural hematoma is low, with an incidence of 1 in 251,463 cases, the complication is difficult to identify and treat.[51] This complication has the potential for catastrophic consequences when bleeding into a fixed space compresses the nerves or spinal cord.[52] Symptoms can develop within 11 to 71 hours after catheter insertion, but the majority occur after 24 hours and include sharp pain in the back or legs progressing to bilateral leg weakness, urinary incontinence, and loss of rectal sphincter tone. Decompression of the hematoma, after diagnosis by computed tomography scan or MRI, is indicated.[53]

A postdural puncture headache results from the leaking of cerebral spinal fluid after dural puncture. The risk is 52.1% after dural puncture with an epidural needle and 1.5% with a spinal needle.[54] Onset of symptoms is usually within 1 to 2 days, but can occur up to 7 days after the incident and can last for 7 days.[54] Symptoms most often include pain in the frontal and occipital areas with radiation to the neck, classically alleviated by remaining in a recumbent position. Severity can be mild to debilitating.[55] A blood patch procedure may alleviate symptoms.[37]

Fetal heart rate abnormalities are a complication of neuraxial anesthesia with a higher incidence after CSE compared with an epidural.[56] Transient fetal bradycardia is most commonly reported and related to increased uterine contractility as a response to decreased plasma epinephrine after swift pain relief once the CSE block is activated.[57]

Von Willebrand's disease is the most common genetic blood dyscrasia. It is classified into subtypes I, II, and III (most severe and least common), based on the level of deficiency of von Willebrand factor. Safety for administration of neuraxial anesthesia is based on the type of vWD, and the degree of deficiency of von Willebrand factor and factor VIII. If coagulation factor levels are normal ($\geq$50 IU/dL), neuraxial anesthesia can be administered safely.[51] If epidural or spinal anesthesia is deemed safe, it should be administered at the request of the woman, using the lowest concentration possible that provides pain relief while also not blocking signs of a neurologic deficit. This principle is particularly important for women who may have either neurologic disease or recent damage owing to injury. These women warrant close monitoring for the signs of hematoma development.[51]

Pregnant women with a history of coagulopathies or an active thrombus/embolus require thromboprophylaxis or therapeutic anticoagulation, respectively. The preferred anticoagulants for parturients are heparin derivatives.[58] To minimize the risk of epidural or spinal hematoma in anticoagulated parturients, women should be transitioned from low-molecular-weight heparin to unfractionated heparin (owing to its shorter half-life) at approximately 36 weeks of gestation.[34] In the event of induction of labor or a planned cesarean birth, low-molecular-weight heparin should be discontinued approximately 24 hours prior.[58] According to the American Society of Regional Anesthesia and Pain Medicine, neuraxial anesthesia should be delayed for 10 to 12 hours after the last prophylactic dose or 24 hours after the last therapeutic dose of low-molecular-weight heparin.[59]

Pregnant women in labor with neurologic conditions such as the existence of, or potential for, elevated ICP (ie, idiopathic intracranial hypertension or secondary intracranial hypertension from an intracranial neoplasm), present a challenge for placement of neuraxial anesthesia owing to the risk of brain stem herniation.[60] Recommendation for or against neuraxial anesthesia will depend on the exact intracranial pathology and whether or not there is an increased risk for disruption between intracranial and spinal canal pressures that leads to increased ICP.[60]

Although pregnancy does not increase the incidence of an intracranial tumor, placental hormones progesterone and estrogen can promote the growth of an existing

Table 4
Local anesthetics: esters and amides

Esters	Amides
2-Chloroprocaine	Lidocaine
Procaine	Bupivacaine
Tetracaine	Ropivacaine

Data from Refs.[37]

Table 5
Local anesthetic modalities

Method	Efficacy/Benefits	Contraindications	Risks
Paracervical block	Injection of a local anesthetic into the vaginal fornix during the first stage of labor to decrease labor pain by blocking the stretch sensation as the cervix dilates.[37,63]	Contraindicated in those with uteroplacental insufficiency or concern for fetal compromise.[37]	Rare. Toxicity can occur from accidental intravascular injection. Parametrial hematoma; paracervical, retropsoas or subgluteal abscess; vasovagal syncope; postpartum neuropathy.[59,60] Fetal toxicity from inadvertent administration into the fetal scalp with transient fetal bradycardia within 10 min after local injection.[59,60,63]
Pudendal nerve block	Transvaginal administration of a local anesthetic injected near the pudendal nerve, using the ischial spines as a landmark.[64] Used for operative birth and/or repair of birth lacerations.	Contraindicated in those who decline or cannot tolerate the procedure, have active bleeding disorders, active vaginal infections, or allergy to a local anesthetic.[64]	Rare. Toxicity from accidental intravascular injection; retroperitoneal hematoma, through damage to a surrounding blood vessel; paracervical, retropsoas or subgluteal abscess.[59,60] Fetal toxicity from inadvertent administration of anesthetic into the fetal scalp.[59,60]
Local infiltration	Injection of an anesthetic into the perineum or affected genital tissue, most commonly used for repair of episiotomy or vaginal laceration.[63]	Contraindicated in those with allergy to local anesthetic.[63]	Fetal toxicity from inadvertent administration of anesthetic into the fetal scalp.[59,60]

Data from Refs.[37,62,63]

lesion.[61] The most common space-occupying lesions (gliomas, meningiomas, and acoustic neuromas) can result in increased ICP.[62] Dural puncture during the administration of neuraxial anesthesia, whether inadvertent during epidural placement or intentional during spinal placement, can result in the loss of cerebral spinal fluid. This leads to a pressure gradient disruption between the intracranium and spina canal, favoring increased ICP, leaving an opportunity for herniation of the brain. Also at great risk for brain herniation are women with evidence of hydrocephalus or increased ICP owing to obstruction of cerebral spinal fluid flow at or above the foramen magnum.[61] In the absence of risk factors suspicious for brain herniation, it may be reasonable to proceed with neuraxial anesthesia in women with known intracranial pathology.[61]

Local Anesthetics (Alternate Regional Analgesic Techniques)

Local anesthetics are either esters or amides.[37] Typically, 1% xylocaine without epinephrine is the choice for injection. Examples of each type are in **Table 4**. Local anesthetic modalities to alleviate pain during childbirth or the repair of perineal lacerations afterward, include the paracervical block, pudendal nerve block, and local tissue infiltration (**Table 5**).

DISCUSSION

Pain and suffering during childbirth are not synonymous and should be interpreted individually by, and with, each woman. There are a multitude of options, both pharmacologic and nonpharmacologic, that may be safely used to alleviate pain in childbirth. For women whose pregnancy is high risk, either from an existing prenatal medical condition or an acute event during labor, the clinician needs to carefully consider the hormonal and physiologic changes of pregnancy, the pain relief modality, any contraindications, efficacy, and maternal wishes when making analgesic and anesthetic decisions. According to the American College of Obstetricians and Gynecologists, the only requirement for administration of neuraxial anesthesia during labor, in the absence of a medical disorder, is maternal request. Via careful consideration of all mediating factors that play into the provision of safe pain relief, the clinician can be assured of providing that which is in the best interest of women and their babies.

REFERENCES

1. Lowe NK. The nature of labor pain. Am J Obstet Gynecol 2002;186:S16–24.
2. Cunningham F, Leveno KJ, Bloom SL, et al. Obstetrical analgesia and anesthesia. In: Cunningham F, Leveno KJ, Bloom SL, et al, editors. Williams obstetrics. 24th edition. New York: McGraw-Hill; 2014. p. 504–22.
3. Hawkins JL. Epidural analgesia for labor and delivery. N Engl J Med 2010; 362(16):1503–10.
4. Priestley W, Storer H, editors. The obstetric memoirs and contributions of James Y. Simpson, MD, FRSE. vol. II. Philadelphia: J.B. Lippincott & Co; 1856.
5. Canton D. Obstetric anesthesia first ten years. Ann Anesth Hist 1970;33(1):102–9.
6. Pitcock CD, Clark RB. From Fanny to Fernand: the development of consumerism in pain control during the birth process. Am J Obstet Gynecol 1992;167(3):581–7.
7. Canton D. The history of obstetric anesthesia. In: Chestnut D, editor. Chestnut's obstetric anesthesia: principles and practice. 5th edition. Philadelphia: Elsevier Saunders; 2014. p. 3–12.
8. Canton D. "In the present state of our knowledge": early use of opioids in obstetrics. Anesthesiology 1995;82(3):779–84.

9. Edwards ML, Jackson AD. The historical development of obstetric anesthesia and its contributions to perinatology. Am J Perinatol 2016;34(3):211–6.

10. Gogarten W, Van Aken H. A century of regional analgesia in obstetrics. Anesth Analg 2000;91(4):773–5.

11. Curelaru I, Sandu L. Eugene Bogdan Aburel (I899-1975): the pioneer of regional analgesia of pain relief in childbirth. Anaesthesia 1982;37:663–9.

12. Charles AG, Norr KL, Block CR, et al. Obstetric and psychological effects of psychoprophylactic preparation for childbirth. Am J Obstet Gynecol 1978;131(1):44–52.

13. Lee SL, Liu CY, Lu YY, et al. Efficacy of warm showers on labor pain and birth experiences during the first labor stage. J Obstet Gynecol Neonatal Nurs 2013;42(1):19–28.

14. Susila DC, Suganthi MS, Tamilarasi B. Effectiveness of hydrotherapy on pain perception during first stage of labour in primi parturient mothers at selected hospital, Chennai. Global J Res Anal 2016;5(6).

15. Taghavi S, Barband S, Khaki A. Effect of hydrotherapy on pain of labor process. Baltica 2015;28(1):116–21.

16. Nutter E, Meyer S, Shaw-Battista J, et al. Waterbirth: an integrative analysis of peer-reviewed literature. J Midwifery Wom Heal 2014;59(3):286–319.

17. Weaver MH. Water birth in the hospital setting. Nurs Womens Health 2014;18(5):365–9.

18. Cluett ER, Burns E. Immersion in water in labour and birth. Cochrane Database Syst Rev 2009;(2):CD000111.

19. Hantoushzadeh S, Alhusseini N, Lebaschi AH. The effects of acupuncture during labour on nulliparous women: a randomised controlled trial. Aust N Z J Obstet Gynaecol 2007;4(1):26–30.

20. Skilnand E, Fossen D, Heiberg E. Acupuncture in the management of pain in labor. Acta Obstet Gynecol Scand 2002;8(10):943–8.

21. Vixner L. Acupuncture for labour pain [Doctoral dissertation]. Stockholm, Sweden: Karolinska Institute; 2015.

22. Vixner L, Schytt E, Stener-Victorin E, et al. Acupuncture with manual and electrical stimulation for labour pain: a longitudinal randomised controlled trial. BMC Complement Altern Med 2014;14(1):187.

23. Dabiri F, Shahi A. The effect of LI4 acupressure on labor pain intensity and duration of labor: a randomized controlled trial. Oman Med J 2014;29(6):425–9.

24. Clarkson CE, O'Mahony D, Jones DE. Adverse event reporting in studies of penetrating acupuncture during pregnancy: a systematic review. Acta Obstet Gynecol Scand 2015;94(5):453–64.

25. Kaviani M, Azima S, Alavi N, et al. The effect of lavender aromatherapy on pain perception and intrapartum outcome in primiparous women. B J Midwifery 2014;22(2):125–8.

26. Namazi M, Akbari AA, Mojab F, et al. Effects of citrus aurantium (Bitter Orange) on the severity of first-stage labor pain. Iran J Pharm Res 2014;13(3):1011–8.

27. Yazdkhasti M, Pirak A. The effect of aromatherapy with lavender essence on severity of labor pain and duration of labor in primiparous women. Complement Ther Clin Pract 2016;25:81–6.

28. Namazi M, Akbari SAA, Mojab F, et al. Aromatherapy with citrus aurantium oil and anxiety during the first stage of labor. Iran Red Crescent 2014;16(6):e18371.

29. Fakari FR, Tabatabaeichehr M, Kamali H, et al. Effect of inhalation of aroma of geranium essence on anxiety and physiological parameters during first stage

of labor in nulliparous women: a randomized clinical trial. J Caring Sci 2015;4(2): 135–41.

30. Fulton KB. Effects of music therapy on physiological measures, perceived pain, and perceived fatigue of women in early labor. [Electronic Theses, Treatises and Dissertation]. Tallahassee (FL): Florida State University; 2005. Paper 4376.

31. Dehcheshmeh FS, Rafiei H. Complementary and alternative therapies to relieve labor pain: a comparative study between music therapy and Hoku point ice massage. Complement Ther Clin Pract 2015;21(4):229–32.

32. Simavli S, Gumus I, Kaygusuz I, et al. Effect of music on labor pain relief, anxiety level and postpartum analgesic requirement: a randomized controlled clinical trial. Gynecol Obstet Invest 2014;78(4):244–50.

33. Manshaee GR, Hemmati M, Karami A. Determining the effectiveness of spiritual therapy on delivery anxiety among 1'st pregnancy women in Imam Ali Hospital, Amol, Iran, 2011. Soc Sci 2016;11(9):2180–8.

34. Blackburn ST. Maternal, fetal, & newborn physiology: a clinical perspective. 4th edition. Maryland Heights (MD): Elsevier; 2013.

35. Canobbio MM, Warnes CA, Aboulhosn J, et al. Management of pregnancy in patients with complex congenital heart disease: a scientific statement for healthcare professional from the American Heart Association. Circulation 2017;135:e1–38.

36. Creasy RK, Resnik R, Iams JD, et al. Maternal-fetal medicine: principles and practice. 7th edition. Philadelphia: Elsevier; 2014.

37. Gabbe SG, Niebyl JR, Simpson JL, et al. Obstetrics. Normal and problem pregnancies. 7th edition. Philadelphia: Elsevier; 2017.

38. Bishop JT. Administration of nitrous oxide in labor: expanding the options for women. J Midwifery Womens Health 2007;52(3):308–9.

39. Starr SA, Collins M, Baysinger C. Vanderbilt University Medical Center Labor and delivery unit policy: nitrous oxide use in the intrapartum/immediate postpartum period (labor and delivery, trans.) (pp. 1–10). Nashville (TN): Vanderbilt University Medical Center; 2011.

40. Stewart L, Collins M. Nitrous oxide as labor analgesia; Clinical implications for nurses. Nurs Womens Health 2012;6(5):398–409.

41. Collins MR, Star SA, Bishop JT, et al. Nitrous oxide for labor analgesia: expanding analgesic options for women in the United States. Rev Obstet Gynecol 2012;5: 3–4.

42. Osterman MJK, Martin J. Epidural and spinal anesthesia use during labor: 27-state reporting area, 2008. Natl Vital Stat Rep 2011;59(5):1–13, 16.

43. Niesen AD, Jacob AK. Combined spinal-epidural versus epidural analgesia for labor and delivery. Clin Perinatol 2013;40(3):373–84.

44. Chestnut DH. Alternative regional analgesic techniques for labor and vaginal delivery. In: Chestnut DH, editor. Chestnut's obstetric anesthesia: principles and practice. 5th edition. Philadelphia: Elsevier Saunders; 2014. p. 518–29.

45. American College of Obstetricians and Gynecologists. Obstetric analgesia and anesthesia. ACOG practice bulletin No. 177. Obstet Gynecol 2017;129:e73–89.

46. Wong C. Epidural and spinal analgesia/anesthesia for labor and vaginal delivery. In: Chestnut D, editor. Chestnut's obstetric anesthesia: principles and practice. 5th edition. Philadelphia: Elsevier Saunders; 2014. p. 457–517.

47. Arko L, Quach E, Nguyen V, et al. Medical and surgical management of spinal epidural abscess: a systematic review. Neurosurg Focus 2014;37(2):E4.

48. Horlocker TT. Complications of regional anesthesia and acute pain management. Anesthesiol Clin 2011;29(2):257–78.

49. Patel AR, Alton TB, Bransford RJ, et al. Spinal epidural abscesses: risk factors, medical versus surgical management, a retrospective review of 128 cases. Spine J 2014;14(2):326–30.
50. Horlocker T, Birnbach D, Connis R, et al. Practice advisory for the prevention, diagnosis, and management of infectious complications associated with neuraxial techniques: a report by the American Society of Anesthesiologists Task Force on infectious complications associated with neuraxial technique. Anesthesiology 2010;112(3):530–45.
51. Gonzalez-Fiol A, Eisenberger A. Anesthesia implications of coagulation and anticoagulation during pregnancy. Semin Perinatol 2014;38(6):370–7.
52. D'Angelo R, Smiley R, Riley E, et al. Serious complications related to obstetric anesthesia. Anesthesiology 2014;120(6):1505–12.
53. Bateman BT, Mhyre JM, Ehrenfeld J, et al. The risk and outcomes of epidural hematomas after perioperative and obstetric epidural catheterization: a report from the multicenter perioperative outcomes group research consortium. Anesth Analg 2013;116(6):1380–5.
54. Choi PT, Galinski SE, Takeuchi L, et al. PDPH is a common complication of neuraxial blockade in parturients: a meta-analysis of obstetrical studies. Can J Anaesth 2003;50(5):460–9.
55. Macarthur A. Postpartum headache. In: Chestnut D, editor. Chestnut's obstetric anesthesia: principles and practice. 5th edition. Philadelphia: Elsevier Saunders; 2014. p. 713–38.
56. Hattler J, Klimek M, Rossaint R, et al. The effect of combined spinal-epidural versus epidural analgesia in laboring women on nonreassuring fetal heart rate tracings: systematic review and meta-analysis. Anesth Analg 2016;123(4):955–64.
57. Abrão KC, Francisco RPV, Miyadahira S, et al. Elevation of uterine basal tone and fetal heart rate abnormalities after labor analgesia: a randomized controlled trial. Obstet Gynecol 2009;113(1):41–7.
58. American College of Obstetrics and Gynecologists. Thromboembolism in pregnancy. Practice bulletin No. 123. Obstet Gynecol 2011;118:718–29 (reaffirmed 2014).
59. Horlocker TT, Wedel DJ, Rowlingson JC, et al. Regional anesthesia in the patient receiving antithrombotic or thrombolytic therapy. Reg Anesth Pain Med 2010; 35(1):64–101.
60. Hopkins AN, Alshaeri T, Akst SA, et al. Neurologic disease with pregnancy and considerations for the obstetric anesthesiologist. Semin Perinatol 2014;38(6):359–69.
61. Anson JA, Vaida S, Giampetro DM, et al. Anesthetic management of labor and delivery in patients with elevated intracranial pressure. Int J Obstet Anesth 2015;24(2):147–60.
62. Leffert L, Schwamm L. Neuraxial anesthesia in parturients with intracranial pathology. Anesthesiology 2013;119(3):703–18.
63. Volmanen P, Palomaki O, Ahonen J. Alternatives to neuraxial analgesia for labor. Curr Opin Anaesthesiol 2011;24(3):235–41.
64. Anderson D. Pudendal nerve block for vaginal birth. J Midwifery Womens Health 2014;(1526):651–9.

Management of Chronic Stable Angina

Michele Ann Walters, DNP, APRN, FNP-BC, CNE

KEYWORDS

- Chronic stable angina • Quality of life • Ischemic heart disease
- Congestive heart failure

KEY POINTS

- Chronic stable angina is diagnosed when symptoms are present for at least 2 months without changes in severity, character, or triggering circumstances.
- Chronic stable angina symptoms are predictable in frequency, severity, duration, and provocation.
- Current treatment strategies are aimed to prevent progression of atherosclerosis, control symptoms, and improve quality of life for the individual.
- Management of chronic stable angina requires a multifaceted treatment modality.

Chronic stable angina (CSA) is a symptomatic problem that is precipitated by ischemic heart disease. Ischemic heart disease, also referred to as coronary heart disease, is diagnosed when there is an inadequate supply of blood to the myocardium.[1] Ischemic heart disease may present as stable or unstable angina. CSA is diagnosed when symptoms are present for at least 2 months without changes in severity, character, or triggering circumstances.[2] CSA is provoked by exertion and relieved by rest because myocardial supply and demand are determinants of the coronary ischemia. CSA symptoms are predictable in frequency, severity, duration, and provocation. The clinical presentation should be evaluated with a detailed history of angina quality, location, radiation, severity, duration, and precipitating and relieving factors. Angina history with associated factors and medications should be elicited from the client (**Table 1**).[2] Current treatment strategies are aimed to prevent progression of atherosclerosis, control symptoms, and improve quality of life for the individual.[2]

Disclosure Statement: There are no relationships with any commercial companies that have a direct financial interest in the subject matter or materials discussed in this article or with any company making a competing product.
Department of Nursing, Morehead State University, St. Claire Regional Family Medicine, 316 West Second Street, CHER 201F, Morehead, KY 40351, USA
E-mail address: ma.walters@moreheadstate.edu

Crit Care Nurs Clin N Am 29 (2017) 487–493
http://dx.doi.org/10.1016/j.cnc.2017.08.008
ccnursing.theclinics.com

Table 1
Angina history

Precipitating factors	Activity related to ADL and walking Meals Stress Cold
Angina Characteristics	Quality of the pain (pressure, stabbing, tightness burning) Radiation (left arm, shoulder, back, neck, jaw) Relief measures (rest, use of nitroglycerin) Severity of pain (rate on numeric pain scale) Timing (activity, times of stress, and note duration of angina event)
Associated Factors	Diaphoresis Dyspnea Paroxysmal nocturnal dyspnea Orthopnea (assess how they sleep: number of pillows or sleeps in a recliner) Gastrointestinal complaints (nausea, vomiting) Fatigue
Medication Profile	Encourage to carry current medication list Review list for medication adherence

Data from Tarkin J, Kaski J. Pharmacological treatment of chronic stable angina pectoris. Clin Med 2013;13(1):63–70.

STRATEGIES TO PREVENT DISEASE PROGRESSION

Management of CSA requires a multifaceted treatment modality. The provider and client's goal should be to slow the ischemic heart disease progression through the ranks of heart failure. Clients should initially undergo noninvasive stress testing and echocardiography to determine left ventricular function.[3] Coronary angiography is appropriate when information from the procedure will significantly influence patient management or if a patient is a candidate for percutaneous coronary intervention (PCI) or surgical revascularization. Current guidelines recommend that optimal medical therapies and lifestyle modification be the first-line treatment of low-risk patients with CSA.[4] In CSA, the choice to pursue PCI is elective. The risks associated with PCI, which include myocardial infarction, restenosis, and death, come with no added benefit of decreased morbidity and mortality in the CSA client.[4]

Optimal medical therapies should include acetylsalicylic acid, beta blockers, calcium channel blockers, lipid-lowering agents, and nitrates as needed.[3] Aspirin therapy doses of 75 mg to 325 mg daily are associated with the best risk–benefit ratio.[1] Clients at risk for gastrointestinal bleeding should be treated with 81 mg per day, plus a proton pump inhibitor. Clopidogrel is an alternative in clients allergic to aspirin.[1] In the client who presents with congestive heart failure with left ventricular ejection fraction (LVEF) less than 40%, the recommendations suggest a renin-angiotensin system inhibition treatment with an angiotensin-converting enzyme (ACE) inhibitor or angiotensin receptor blocker (ARB), or an angiotensin receptor neprilysin inhibitor (ARNI).[5] ARNI is a combination of an ARB with an inhibitor of neprilysin (valsartan-sacubitril), which is an enzyme that degrades natriuretic peptides, bradykinin, adrenomedullin, and other vasoactive peptides.[5] In random controlled trials, ARNI reduced cardiovascular death and heart failure hospitalizations. The client taking ARNI should be monitored for hypotension, renal insufficiency, and angioedema.

STRATEGIES TO CONTROL ANGINA SYMPTOMS

In patients with CSA, the occurrence of equal to or greater than 1 episode of angina on a weekly basis is associated with worse quality of life and greater physical limitations.[6] The 3 traditional classes of anti-ischemic drugs commonly used in the management of angina are beta blockers, calcium channel blockers, and nitrates.[1] When a combination of these traditional therapies and long-acting nitrates do not achieve the expectations of the client, the provider may look for other alternatives for angina control. Recommendations for ivabradine can be beneficial to reduce heart failure hospitalization and has shown to improve quality of life by decreasing episodes of angina.[5,7] Ivabradine should be considered in clients with LVEF less than 35%, receiving a beta blocker at the maximum tolerated dose, and in normal sinus rhythm with a resting heart rate of equal to or greater than 70 beats per minute.[5] Ivabradine's mechanism of action blocks the hyperpolarization-activated cyclic nucleotide-gated channel responsible for the cardiac pacemaker I_f current, which regulates heart rate.[8] Ivabradine can also inhibit the retinal current I_h responsible for the luminous phenomena or a visual halo effect. Other adverse reactions to ivabradine include bradycardia, hypertension, and atrial fibrillation.

Another consideration for control of CSA is the sodium channel inhibitor ranolazine. Ranolazine has been found to decrease angina and increase activity tolerance.[6,9] Ranolazine may be used in combination with beta-blockers, calcium channel blockers, renin-angiotensin system inhibitors, lipid-lowering therapy, and nitrates.[10] The mechanism of action of ranolazine has not been determined. However, the anti-ischemic and antianginal effects do not depend on reductions in heart rate or blood pressure. Ranolazine blocks I_{kr} and prolongs the QTc interval. The client with diabetes may benefit from ranolazine because a small reduction in hemoglobin A1c was noted with the use of the medication during clinical trials. The client taking metformin for their diabetes should be limited to 1700 mg daily because ranolazine will increase plasma levels of metformin.[10]

As a provider, it is a difficult task to determine which pharmacologic agent is best for a client. One study compared the efficacy and tolerability of ivabradine and ranolazine.[11] The study concluded that both medications were equal as antianginals but the ranolazine appeared superior by tolerability by the client, demonstrated a better safety profile, and was found to be more cost-effective than the ivabradine.[11]

The most widely accepted option for angina control is sublingual nitroglycerin. The use of sublingual nitroglycerin spray before exercise has demonstrated increased time before onset of moderate angina during exercise.[12] It is recommended that clients use the sublingual nitroglycerin spray prophylactically before exercise to minimize angina. Nitrate tolerance is a major limitation to continuous nitrate therapy.[3] Nitrate-free intervals of at a minimum of 8 hours daily should be encouraged to minimize nitrate tolerance. There are multiple nitrate preparations available to the client in short-acting and long-acting preparations (**Table 2**).[13] Clients should be educated on prophylactic use of short-acting nitroglycerin preparations in activities that precipitate angina, such as mowing the lawn, shoveling snow, or walking in cold weather. Prophylactic use of nitroglycerin is not sufficiently emphasized to clients, therefore education should be provided at multiple primary care visits.[1] When prescribed nitroglycerin, the client should receive education regarding proper storage regarding heat and photosensitivity of the medication. The provider should include instructions for the client taking short-acting nitroglycerin to sit down when initiating the medication to prevent orthostatic hypotension and syncopal episodes.

Chronic nitrate therapy is used to prevent recurrent angina episodes but must be dosed correctly to prevent tolerance. Long-acting nitrates should be prescribed for

Table 2
Nitrate preparations

Preparation	Starting Dose	Maximum Dose	Onset of Action
Nitroglycerin (Nitrostat)	0.4 mg tablet	3 tablets in 15 min	1 min
Nitroglycerin (Nitrolingual)	0.4 mg (metered spray)	3 sprays in 15 min	1 min
Nitroglycerin Powder packet (GoNitro)	400mcg powder packet	3 packets within 15 min	1 min
Isosorbide dinitrate	10–40 mg bid Extended-release form 40 mg daily	480 mg/d Extended-release form 160 mg/d	30–60 min
Isosorbide mononitrate	Immediate-release form 20 mg bid Extended-release form 30 mg, 60 mg, 120 mg daily	Immediate-release form 40 mg/d Extended-release form 240 mg/d	30–60 min
Nitroglycerin topical (Nitro-Bid 2% ointment)	0.5 in every 4–6 h	2–5 in topical every 4 h	30–60 min
Nitroglycerin transdermal patch 0.1, 0.2, 0.4, 0.6 mg/h	1 patch daily for 12–14 h then off for 10–12 h	1 patch in 14 h	24 h

Data from Vallerand A, Sanoski C. Davis's drug guide for nurses. 15th edition. Philadelphia: F.A. Davis Company; 2017.

angina symptoms when monotherapy with beta blockers is no longer effective, or they may be used as monotherapy if there are contraindications to beta blockers.[1]

Nonconventional angina therapy being researched is the supplementation of vitamin D. Vitamin D deficiency is associated with vascular endothelial dysfunction, which leads to atherosclerosis and coronary artery disease (CAD).[14,15] Research conducted by Sagarad and colleagues[15] identified a significant reduction in angina episodes and a decreased use of sublingual nitroglycerine after vitamin D supplementation. Clients in the research study were provided 60,000 IU of vitamin D supplementation every week for 8 weeks. There was a significant decrease in frequency of angina episodes (20%) and use of sublingual nitroglycerine (17%) from baseline.[15] Raina and colleagues[16] support the correlation between vitamin D deficiency and CSA. Rania and colleagues[16] identified that smokers will have lower vitamin D levels than nonsmokers. Although there has not been a large controlled study conducted regarding vitamin D therapy, there is sufficient evidence to consider screening a client with CSA for vitamin D insufficiency and to consider vitamin D_3 replacement therapy.

QUALITY OF LIFE

There has been a considerable amount of research into the illness representation of cardiac clients. Negative illness perceptions have been associated with reduced quality of life, medical complications, delayed returned to work, reduced lifestyle, and cardiac rehabilitation attendance.[17] The first step toward successful treatment of a client with CSA is an effective evaluation of angina severity and its impact on quality of life.[18] Multiple screening tools are available. An example of a screening tool for angina is provided in **Box 1**. "Speak from the Heart Chronic Angina Checklist,"

Box 1
Chronic angina checklist

1. In the past month, how many times have you had angina?
   None
   1 to 4
   5 to 8
   9 or more

2. Have you cut back or totally given up any activities or work because of your angina?
   Yes
   No
   If so, what?

3. Do you ever have angina while
   Feeling stressed
   Having sex
   In hot or cold weather
   Resting
   Dressing
   Bathing
   Walking at an ordinary pace
   Climbing stairs
   Other times

4. How much has angina affected your quality of life?
   Not at all
   A little
   Somewhat
   A lot
   Very much

5. Has angina affected your family life?
   Yes
   No
   If so, how?

6. Is there anything else you would like to talk with your doctor about? (Check all that apply.)
   Treatment side effects
   Diet and exercise
   Other

Data from Gilead sciences. "The speak from the heart chronic angina checklist," Web site 2016. Available at: http://www.speakfromtheheart.com/angina-tools/angina-tracker. Accessed April 27, 2017.

which is available online to download for clients, assists clients in tracking their symptoms on a calendar.[19]

Once screening has taken place for the impact that the angina has on the client's quality of life. The American Heart Association recommends screening for depressive symptoms in clients with established coronary heart disease.[20] There are no specific depression screening scales for individuals with coronary heart disease or congestive heart failure but there are suspected cardiotoxic psychological symptoms in clients with CAD.[21] If depression is identified, sertraline has the best safety profile reported for cardiac clients.[20] Tricyclic antidepressants should be avoided because they can cause QT prolongation and lead to arrhythmic deaths.

The association with depression and lower exercise capacity and quality of life is complicated, which suggests that there are other variables that interfere with a client's functional capacity with CAD. Bunevicius and colleagues[21] identify that differences in personality traits may have an adverse effect on these outcomes. The type D personality is a combination of a negative affectivity (tendency to experience negative emotions) and tendency to inhibit self-expression, which are symptoms of fatigue and mental distress in a cardiac client. Type D personalities are associated with adverse clinical events and poor health status. Type D personalities are less motivated to engage in physical activity; therefore they may not fully participate in cardiac rehabilitation efforts. They are also more likely to suffer from depressive symptoms. Identifying type D personalities earlier is an area that needs more research.

In summary, the management of CSA to maximize one's quality of life is complex. The American Heart Association recommends that all clients with stable ischemic heart disease receive education and counseling regarding medication compliance, controlling risk factors, and regular exercise.[1] Controlling risk factors may include education about and treatment of hypertension, smoking cessation, initiation of statin therapy, weight reduction, and monitoring glycemic control.[1] Exercise programs should be encouraged with a recommendation for a referral to participate in cardiac rehabilitation programs. All clients with ischemic heart disease should receive an annual influenza vaccine.[1] Clients should be encouraged to keep regular follow-up visits with their primary care provider every 6 to 12 months to discuss changes in physical activity and angina frequency or severity, monitor for new or worsening of comorbid illnesses, assess for tolerance of medication, and verify medication adherence.[1] The visit should consist of laboratory evaluations for diabetes and hyperlipidemia, and monitoring for electrocardiogram changes. Although CSA can be complicated to manage, the client need not feel alone. Clinicians should encourage clients to be active in their own care by connecting with social networks and professional organizations sponsored by local, state, and national associations.

REFERENCES

1. Kannam J, Aroesty J, Gersh B, et al. Stable ishchemic hear disease: overview of care. UpToDate 2017. Available at: http://www.uptodate.com. Accessed April 27, 2017.
2. Tarkin J, Kaski J. Pharmacological treatment of chronic stable angina pectoris. Clin Med 2013;13(1):63–70.
3. Buttaro T, Tyrbulski J, Polgar-Bailey P, et al. Primary care: a collaborative practice. 5th edition. St Louis (MO): Elsevier; 2017. p. 540.
4. Behnke L, Solis A, Shulman S, et al. A targeted approach to reducing overutilization: use of percutaneous coronary intervention in stable coronary artery disease. Popul Health Manag 2013;16(3):164–8.
5. Yancy CW, Jessup M, Bozkurt B, et al. 2016 ACC/AHA/AFSA focused update on new pharmacological therapy for heart failure; an update of the 2013 ACF/AHA guideline for the management of heart failure; a report of the American College of Cardiology/American Heart Association Task Force on Clinical Practice Guidelines and the Heart Failure Society of America. Circulation 2016;134:e282–93.
6. Muhlestein J, Grehan S. Ranolazine reduces patient-reported angina severity and frequency and improves quality of life in selected patients with chronic angina. J Pharmacol Pharmacother 2017;8(1):207–13.
7. Zanky H, Elzein H, Alsheikh-Ali A, et al. Short-term effects of Ivabradine in patients with chronic stable ischemic heart disease. Heart Views 2013;2(14):53–5.
8. Full prescribing information. Corlanor Web site 2017. Available at: http://www.corlanorhcp.com. Accessed April 24, 2017.

9. Keating G. Ranolazine: a review of its use as add-on therapy in patients with chronic stable angina pectoris. Drugs 2013;73:55–73.
10. Full prescribing information. Ranexa Web site 2017. Available at: http://www.ranexahcp.com. Accessed April 25, 2017.
11. Chaturvedi A, Yogendra S, Chaturvedi H, et al. Comparison of the efficacy and tolerability of ivabradine and ranolazine in patients of chronic stable angina pectoris. J Pharmacol Pharmacother 2013;4(1):33–7.
12. Thadani U, Wittig T. A randomized, double-blind, placebo-controlled, crossover, dose-ranging multicenter study to determine the effect of sublingual nitroglycerin spray on exercise capacity in patients with chronic stable angina. Clin Med Insights Cardiol 2012;6:87–95.
13. Vallerand A, Sanoski C. Davis's drug guide for nurses. 15th edition. Philadelphia: F.A. Davis Company; 2017.
14. Hashemi S, Mokhtari S, Sadeghi M, et al. Effect of vitamin D therapy on endothelial function in ischemic heart disease female patients with vitamin D deficiency or insufficiency: a primary report. ARYA Atheroscler 2015;11(1):54–9.
15. Sagarad S, Sukhani N, Machanur B, et al. Effect of vitamin D on angina episodes in vitamin d deficient patients with chronic stable angina on medical management. J Clin Diagn Res 2016;10(8):24–6.
16. Raina A, Allai M, Shah Z, et al. Association of low levels of vitamin D with chronic stable angina: a prospective case-control study. N Am J Med Sci 2016;8:143–50.
17. Le Grande M, Elliott P, Worcester M, et al. Identifying illness perceptions schemata and their association with depression and quality of life in cardiac patients. Psychol Health Med 2012;17(6):709–22.
18. Young J Jr, Melander S. Evaluating symptoms to improve quality of life in patients with chronic stable angina. Nurs Res Pract 2013;2013:504915.
19. Gilead sciences. "The speak from the heart chronic angina checklist," Web site 2016. Available at: http://www.speakfromtheheart.com/angina-tools/angina-tracker. Accessed April 27, 2017.
20. Tofler G. Psychosocial factors in acute myocardial infaction. UpToDate 2017. Available at: http://www.uptodate.com. Accessed April 27, 2017.
21. Bunevicius A, Brozaitiene J, Staniute M, et al. Decreased physical effort, fatigue, and mental distress in patients with coronary artery disease: importance of personality-related differences. Int J Behav Med 2014;21:240–7.

The Use of Remifentanil as the Primary Agent for Analgesia in Parturients

Bryan Anderson, DNAP, CRNA

KEYWORDS

- Ultiva • Remifentanil • Obstetric analgesia • Analgesia in parturients
- Opioids in pregnancy

KEY POINTS

- In parturients desiring analgesia for labor, there are limited alternatives to neuraxial anesthesia techniques. Remifentanil is an alternative.
- The significance of remifentanil use as the primary analgesic in parturients for whom neuraxial anesthesia is not an option is explored in detail.
- Recommendations regarding the use of remifentanil for labor pain can provide safe anesthesia delivery while enhancing the provision of care to parturients.

To achieve optimal patient outcomes in anesthesia patients, it is important to consider multiple options for pain control, especially when traditional options pose a problem or are not options. In particular, there are parturient clients for whom the use of neuraxial anesthesia (epidural and spinal blockade) is not an option. In these cases, an alternative option that warrants consideration for patient centered anesthesia practice is the use of remifentanil (Ultiva). Guidelines for the use of remifentanil in obstetric patients are sparse, poorly developed, and not readily available to anesthesia practitioners.

PAIN ASSOCIATED WITH LABOR

There is no question about the amount and extent of pain associated with child birth. There are some common interventions used to ameliorate pain, including the use of epidural anesthesia. However, there are several reasons that an epidural may be contraindicated during labor, including the presence of coagulopathies, anticoagulation therapy, prior back surgery, patient refusal, or the inability to safely place an epidural. In labor patients for whom neuraxial anesthesia is not an option, there are limited alternative choices that have been explored or considered. Once such possibility deserving of consideration is the use of the opioid remifentanil as the primary analgesic for the management of pain associated with labor.

Middle Tennessee School of Anesthesia, 315 Hospital Drive, Madison, TN 37115, USA
E-mail address: banderson@mtsa.edu

Crit Care Nurs Clin N Am 29 (2017) 495–517
http://dx.doi.org/10.1016/j.cnc.2017.08.009
0899-5885/17/© 2017 Elsevier Inc. All rights reserved.

ccnursing.theclinics.com

Olufolabi and colleagues[1] identified "that the cyclical pattern of labor pain, as compared with continuous postoperative surgical pain, would benefit from bolus delivery of a short-acting drug that produced its analgesic effect only during contractions and was without significant maternal and fetal side effects." One such drug that should be considered is remifentanil.

THE IMPORTANCE OF EXPLORING REMIFENTANIL AS AN OPTION FOR TREATING LABOR PAIN

The use of remifentanil in the parturient as the primary analgesic is significant for several reasons, the most salient of which is the basic human right to the management of pain. Pain, as defined by the International Association for the Study of Pain, is "an unpleasant sensory and emotional experience associated with actual or potential tissue damage."[2] Labor is a cause of severe pain for many women and is a problem that should be addressed and managed in accordance with the needs and wishes of the individual patient. Interventions that alleviate or eliminate pain are not merely a matter of beneficence, but also form part of the duty to prevent harm.[3]

The variations in pain perception among women in labor creates an essential component in the administration of anesthesia in the provision of patient-centered anesthesia care. One recent study identifies that the perception of labor pain was equivalent to a digit amputation without anesthesia.[4] Even though variability regarding the intensity of pain exists among women during labor, the majority of women do experience more than minimal pain during this time.[5] Negative psychological effects of pain associated with labor can occur in some women. "Psychological harm can be experienced through the provision or withholding of labor analgesia, underscoring the tremendous variability in the meaning of labor pain for different women."[5] Interventions to alleviate pain in labor have effects on much more than the physical aspects of pain, but also include the emotional and psychological factors.

Epidural analgesia is considered the standard for pain management during labor.[5] Access to pain management is a right that is fundamental and should not be withheld or denied to any patient regardless of age, ethnicity, or socioeconomic status. This right is violated if a parturient is unable to partake in standard methods used for managing the pain of labor. The significance of analgesia during labor is related to the access parturients have to care. "Equity is concerned with maximizing fairness in the distribution of healthcare services...and minimizing disparities in health."[6] By using an intervention such as remifentanil, the alleviation of pain associated with labor encompasses a greater portion of this population.

A patient's perception of their analgesic regimen is also a concern. It is central for a provider to address this intervention that is rooted in reliable evidence. The use of patient-controlled analgesia (PCA) puts the patient in control when dosing of medication occurs and is considered the gold standard for acute pain management.[7] Patient satisfaction with remifentanil as a primary analgesic for labor pain is an important topic within this context. There is evidence that maternal satisfaction is influenced by factors other than age, ethnicity, socioeconomic status, pain, medical interventions, and continuity of care, when women evaluate their childbirth experiences. These overriding factors have been identified as personal expectations, the amount of support from caregivers, quality of the caregiver–patient relationship, and maternal involvement in decision making. The results of pain, pain relief, and intrapartum medical interventions on the satisfaction of parturients are not as obvious, direct, or powerful as the influences and impact of the attitudes and behaviors of caregivers.[8]

To provide optimal anesthesia care to clients, the body of knowledge on which evidence-based practice is founded must continue to evolve as new information and research comes to light.[9] Certified Registered Nurse Anesthetists (CRNAs) have been recognized as influential providers in the area of pain management, because the knowledge and skills possessed required to address this issue are essential to the study and understanding of acute and chronic pain.[10] Reviewing the current evidence related to the use of remifentanil as a primary agent for analgesia in parturients enables the CRNA to make a recommendation or construct a set of guidelines that may be used in clinical practice. This recommendation or guideline can provide a basis for knowledge and safety of anesthesia delivery while enhancing the provision of care to parturients.

FOUNDATIONAL PRINCIPLES

Understanding the underlying physiology of pain associated with labor, and the pharmacokinetics and pharmacology of remifentanil, is an essential for the CRNA to effectively and safely provide efficient anesthesia interventions. The pain associated with labor is highly personal and varies greatly among individual patients.[5,10] There are 3 stages of labor that must be considered when discussing the physiologic basis for pain related to each. The first stage of labor has 2 phases—latent and active—and is defined as the onset of labor, which progresses to the complete dilation of the cervix. The second stage of labor begins when the cervix is fully dilated (10 cm), and ends when delivery of the infant is complete. The third stage occurs with delivery of the placenta.[10] For purposes here, only the first and second stages are considered.

Pain of Labor

Labor can be defined as progressive dilatation of the cervix in association with repetitive uterine contractions.[11] The pain of labor arises from several sources. These include contraction of the myometrium against the resistance of the cervix and perineum, progressive dilatation of the cervix and lower uterine segment, and stretching and compression of pelvic and perineal structures. Two manifestations of pain have been identified by parturients. They are a nonlocalized cramping, which is referred to surface dermatomes on the abdomen and sharp, and localized back pain that is from referred pain to dermatomes and sclerotomes.[10] Each stage of labor has different origins and pathways.

Pain during the first stage of labor is mostly visceral pain resulting from uterine contractions and cervical dilatation.[12] This pain is mediated by T10 to L1 sympathetic nerve fibers, and the nerves at this level are responsible for transmitting pain sensation related to cervical dilation.[10] In the first stage of labor, pain is initially confined to the T11 and T12 dermatomes during the latent phase, but eventually involves the T10 to L1 dermatomes as the labor enters the active phase. Parturients describe this pain as dull in nature and often poorly localized.[11] The visceral afferent fibers responsible for labor pain travel with sympathetic nerve fibers, first to the uterine and cervical plexuses, then through the hypogastric and aortic plexuses before entering the spinal cord with the T10 to L1 nerve roots.[12]

The second stage of labor is entered as cervical dilation becomes complete and fetal descent begins. During this stage, pain is transmitted by the same afferent nerves activated during the first stage of labor (T10–L1) with the addition of nerves at the S1 to S4 levels. These nerves of the sacral plexus innervate the cervix, vagina, and perineum.[5,10] Compression and stretching of muscles and ligaments in the pelvic region produce pain that is mediated by the sacral plexus.[10] This stretching and compression of perineal structures may intensify pain.[12]

Pharmacology of Remifentanil

In addition to an understanding the physiology of pain in labor, the pharmacology of the drug in question—remifentanil—must also be considered. Remifentanil is a selective mu (μ) agonist similar in potency to fentanyl. Its ester linkage makes remifentanil structurally unique and renders the drug susceptible to hydrolysis by nonspecific plasma and tissue esterases to metabolites that are inactive. The onset and duration of action for remifentanil are very short, making it rapidly titratable. Effect site (blood–brain) equilibration time is 1.1 minutes and elimination half-time is 6 minutes. An estimated 99.8% of remifentanil is eliminated during the distribution (0.9 minute) and elimination (6 minutes) half-time.[12] This short duration of action and minimal accumulation with repeated doses or infusion make remifentanil particularly well-suited for procedures that are briefly painful but for which little postoperative analgesia is required.[13]

The pharmacokinetics of remifentanil are characterized by a small volume of distribution (30 L), rapid clearance, and low interindividual variability as compared with other drugs. Rapid effect-site equilibration equates to a quickly achieved steady state plasma and effect-site concentration. Additionally, the plasma concentration is nearly independent of infusion duration owing to the short, context-sensitive half-time. Changes in infusion rates of remifentanil are paralleled by prompt changes in drug effect. These attributes make the pharmacokinetics similar in obese and lean patients. Owing to the low interindividual variability, it is recommended that clinical dosing regimens be based on ideal body mass and not total body weight.[14]

Metabolism by nonspecific plasma and tissue esterases to inactive metabolites make remifentanil unique. The principal metabolite is remifentanil acid, which is 300 to 4600 times less potent than the parent drug. Excretion is primarily via renal pathways and it is unlikely that the pharmacokinetics are changed in the presence of renal or hepatic failure because esterase metabolism is usually preserved in these states.[14] Esterase metabolism has little variability between individuals and contributes greatly to the predictability of drug effect. Minimal changes are related to extremes of age, renal dysfunction, or hepatic dysfunction, enabling easy titration and rapid dissipation, even after prolonged infusion.[15]

Adverse effects resulting from the administration of remifentanil are similar to those of any other potent opioids.[16] These include, but are not limited to, lightheadedness, dyspnea, blurred vision, chest pain, and muscle stiffness or tightness. With remifentanil use, profound analgesia may be achieved with minimal effect on cognitive function, and low doses of remifentanil can be used to maintain anesthesia in spontaneously breathing patients.[15,17]

Remifentanil is licensed for induction and maintenance of general anesthesia; however, it is currently an off-label use in obstetrics.[17] Even though remifentanil is not licensed for use in obstetric patients, the administration of drugs outside their product license is a common occurrence in obstetric anesthesia.[18]

CONDITIONS IN WHICH STANDARD NEURAXIAL ANESTHESIA IS A NONOPTION

Several factors must be considered when discussing the use of neuraxial anesthesia for labor analgesia. These include generally recognized absolute and relative contraindications for neuraxial anesthesia, such as bleeding or clotting disorders (coagulopathies), severe hypovolemia, elevated intracranial pressure, valvular heart disease, infection at the injection site, or patient refusal.[10] Additional factors include anticoagulation therapy, prior back surgery, or the inability to perform a neuraxial anesthetic. This discussion is not intended to be all inclusive, but rather to highlight several clinically relevant factors regarding the subject of neuraxial anesthesia being a nonoption for some parturients.

The existence of coagulopathies in a patient may be preexisting or therapeutic in nature. Frank coagulopathies represent an absolute contraindication to the administration of neuraxial anesthesia. Concern with performing neuraxial anesthesia in parturients with coagulopathy is due to an increased risk of epidural hematoma formation.[5] The incidence of occurrence is rare, but the resultant neurologic damage may be permanent.[10]

Thrombocytopenia is an intrinsic coagulopathy that is defined as a platelet count of less than 100,000/mm^3. The use of neuraxial anesthesia is generally not recommended for parturients with platelet counts of less than 100,000/mm^3; however, some practitioners may have a lower cutoff.[10] One disorder involving thrombocytopenia that may be encountered in the parturient is autoimmune thrombocytopenic purpura. In autoimmune thrombocytopenic purpura, antibodies directed against platelet antigens are produced primarily in the spleen, where phagocytosis by macrophages occurs.[5] This destruction of platelets leads to decreased platelet counts and an increased risk for bleeding. The anesthesia provider should consider clinical evidence of bleeding, recent platelet count, a recent change in platelet count, quality of platelets, adequacy of other coagulation factors, and the risks versus the benefits of performing neuraxial anesthesia. It is important to note that "clinical judgment represents the most important means of assessing the risk for epidural hematoma in an individual patient."[5]

It is important to consider the impact of anticoagulation therapy in the parturient because this poses a contraction to traditional neuraxial anesthesia. The use of unfractionated heparin and low-molecular-weight heparin may be encountered in the parturient being treated for coagulopathic states such as thrombotic thrombocytopenic purpura and disseminated intravascular coagulation. The American Society of Regional Anesthesia and Pain Medicine guidelines are specific regarding neuraxial anesthesia in the presence of anticoagulant use.[18] For the parturient receiving intravenous (IV) heparin, there should be at least a 1-hour delay between needle placement and heparin administration.[19] The safety of neuraxial blockade in patients receiving doses greater than 10,000 units of unfractionated heparin daily, or more than twice daily dosing of unfractionated heparin, has not been established. Protamine reversal of heparin therapy to allow administration of neuraxial anesthesia is not recommended.[5] For parturients who are receiving treatment with the low-molecular-weight heparin enoxaparin, neuraxial anesthesia should be performed at least 12 hours after the last prophylactic dose or 24 hours after higher doses (1 mg/kg every 12 hours).[19] Parturients receiving anticoagulation therapy may be excluded from the benefits of neuraxial anesthesia.

Skeletal deformities such as scoliosis, arthritis, osteoporosis, and fusion or scarring of the vertebrae are relative contraindications to neuraxial anesthesia. Needle placement may be difficult and the spread of medications in the epidural space may be limited by these anatomic alterations.[10] Guidelines for epidural anesthesia after spinal surgery are not clearly defined.[20] Posterior approach surgical techniques often obliterate or distort the epidural space from fibrous scar tissue formation, blood clot organization, or metalwork crossing the midline.[20] Combined with the fact that anatomic landmarks for neuraxial anesthesia may be difficult to assess, regardless of the parturient's history of corrective surgery, this approach to pain management is one that requires careful scrutiny. The disadvantages of neuraxial anesthesia include technical difficulties in identifying the epidural space, patchy or poor analgesia, unintentional subdural or intrathecal catheter placement, and postdural puncture headache.[21] Both parturients and anesthesia providers may be willing to attempt neuraxial anesthesia in these situations; however, the risks versus the benefit must be understood and accepted by all parties.

Parturients with severe, uncorrected hypovolemia are considered to have a relative contraindication to neuraxial anesthesia.[10] Severe hypovolemia can precipitate a vagal response that results in profound bradycardia, or possibly transient cardiac arrest in patients who are healthy. Bradycardia is mediated by left ventricular mechanoreceptors, which are activated by a decrease in venous return and the resulting reduction of end-systolic volume.[22] It is recommended that epidural blockade be used with great care or even avoided in patients with hypovolemia in whom venous return is impaired.[22]

The use of neuraxial techniques always presents a risk of dural puncture with an epidural needle. Puncture of the dura may create a hole in the dural tissue and subsequent cerebrospinal fluid leak. Patients with elevated intracranial pressure have an increased risk for brain herniation. Epidural catheter placement and addition of large volumes of local anesthetic may cause an increase in already elevated intracranial pressures.[10]

The presence of valvular heart disease, such as idiopathic hypertrophic subaortic stenosis or other fixed volume cardiac states, are a relative contraindication to neuraxial anesthesia when considered clinically mild to moderate in severity. Neuraxial techniques are contraindicated in patients with severe cardiac disease.[12] Physiologic changes such as bradycardia, decreased systemic vascular resistance, and decreased venous return are all changes that can be encountered with neuraxial anesthesia. These physiologic changes are not tolerated and may cause hypotension that results in severe coronary hypoperfusion and cardiac arrest.[10,12] Each patient requires evaluation, and the risks versus the benefit must be understood and accepted by all parties if the implementation of a neuraxial technique is considered.

Infection at the site of needle placement for neuraxial anesthesia is a concern owing to the risk of disrupting the body's physiologic protection mechanisms. The epidural needle may deposit infectious or noxious agents beyond the skin into the underlying tissue, peridural space, and past the blood–brain barrier into the subarachnoid space.[10] The use of neuraxial anesthesia in the presence of sepsis or bacteremia may dispose a parturient to the spread of the infectious agents into the epidural or subarachnoid space and increase the risk for meningitis or the formation of an epidural abscess.[10,12] These risks make neuraxial anesthesia an absolute contraindication in the presence of infection at the needle site.

The most compelling contradiction for not using neuraxial anesthesia is patient refusal. Parturients may have concerns related to neuraxial anesthesia, including potential for short- or long-term complications, fear of pain with implementation, fear of numbness or altered sensation, lack of control over the anesthetic, or the inability to obtain adequate anesthesia. Proper preparation, education, and collaboration are keys to successful interaction with patients.[10] In cases where a parturient declines the use of neuraxial anesthesia techniques, the provider must be prepared to offer an alternative for managing the pain associated with labor. Alternatives provide access to pain management, and uphold the fundamental right that pain management should not be withheld or denied to any patient.[3]

Remifentanil in Clinical Practice

The literature that compiled and reviewed in the most current studies (metaanalysis, systematic review, reviews of literature, and focused review) revealed that the use of remifentanil as a primary analgesic for the management of labor pain is an accepted practice. When implemented appropriately (regardless of methodology), it is more effective than IV meperidine but less effective than an epidural.[23–26] A 2010 Cochrane Review investigated different parenteral opioids for maternal pain relief during labor and concluded that there is insufficient evidence to identify the best opioid for pain relief[27] (**Table 1**).

Table 1		
An overview of remifentanil		
Classification and metabolism	Intravenous opioid with rapid onset and brief duration. Regulated as a schedule II substance	The brief duration results from rapid metabolism by plasma and tissue esterases, and not from hepatic metabolism or renal excretion.
Potency	100 times more potent than morphine.	Fentanyl is also 100 times more potent than morphine.
Administration and duration	Administered via continuous intravenous infusion	Effects begin in minutes and end 5–10 min once stopped.
Common dose	*For surgical anesthesia:* 0.05–2 µg/kg/min (current evidence varies)	*For postoperative anesthesia* 0.025–0.2 µg/kg/min (current evidence varies)
Adverse effects	*During infusion:* respiratory depression, hypotension, bradycardia, and muscle rigidity sufficient to compromise breathing	*After infusion:* nausea (44%), vomiting (22%), and headache (18%).

Adapted from Lehner RA. Pharmacology for nursing care. 8th edition. St Louis (MO): Elsevier; 2013.

In a 2012 metaanalysis by Schnabel and colleagues[23] evaluating the efficacy of remifentanil PCA compared with other techniques for labor analgesia, 12 randomized, controlled trials with a total of 593 participants, 269 of which received remifentanil, were included. Of the 12 trials in the metaanalysis, healthy term parturients (American Society of Anesthesiologists classification I and II) without a history of opioid use, drug abuse, allergy to remifentanil, or abnormal hepatic or renal function were included. Four different active comparators were investigated—meperidine, fentanyl, nitrous oxide, and epidural analgesia. Owing to limited data, the authors were only able to pool data for the comparison between remifentanil and either meperidine or epidural analgesia.

Eight trials compared remifentanil with meperidine in this metaanalysis; 208 parturients received a remifentanil PCA and 209 received meperidine either via PCA, as a continuous infusion, or as an intramuscular injection. In all 8 of the trials, patients receiving remifentanil had a lower mean pain score after 1 hour compared with patients receiving meperidine (mean difference, −2.17 cm; 95% CI, −2.7 to −1.64; P<.001). Five trials found that women had significantly higher satisfaction scores if they received remifentanil but, because all trials used different scores for maternal satisfaction, these results could not be pooled and were reported only qualitatively.[23]

Three trials investigated the efficacy of a remifentanil PCA in comparison with an epidural; 51 parturients received remifentanil and 51 received an epidural. In all of the included trials, women in the remifentanil group had a higher mean pain relief score after 1 hour compared with the epidural group (mean difference, 1.89 cm; 95% CI, 0.63–3.15; P = .003). Satisfaction scores with the analgesic regimens were comparable.[23]

The conclusions supported in this metaanalysis indicated that remifentanil provided better analgesia than IV or intramuscular meperidine and that epidural analgesia provided better pain relief than remifentanil during labor. It was recommended that large, randomized, controlled trials with a focus on safety and patient satisfaction using consistent administration methods be conducted.[23] In this metaanalysis, the authors failed to find sufficient evidence for dosing regimens and no clinical recommendations regarding dosing or implementation were presented.

A 2011 systematic review by Leong and colleagues[24] comparing remifentanil and meperidine for labor analgesia included 7 studies with a total of 349 patients; however, only 3 studies were suitable for quantitative synthesis in a metaanalysis (233 total patients). The review was performed using a previously specified protocol outlining the aim, search strategy, eligibility criteria, data extraction strategy, and statistical analysis methods to be used. The authors assessed for adequacy of sequence generation, allocation sequence concealment, blinding, and the completeness of follow-up. For studies that were judged to be at higher risk of bias, a sensitivity analysis was performed to assess whether the inclusion of these studies significantly biased the result. The primary outcome was pain scores assessed using a 0 to 100 mm visual analog scale (VAS).

All 7 studies measured the pain scores using a 0- to 100-mm VAS scale; however, only 3 studies were included in the metaanalysis. Three studies were excluded because the VAS data were presented graphically and a fourth study was excluded because pain scores were presented using median and interquartile ranges. The authors noted that all 4 excluded studies found a significant reduction in VAS scores with remifentanil compared with meperidine ($P<.05$, which establishes statistical significance). The results of the 3 studies that reported using the means and standard deviations of VAS scores were quantitatively combined and it was shown that there was a reduction of mean VAS score at 1 hour of 25 mm for remifentanil compared with meperidine ($P<.001$; 95% CI, 19–31 mm). When all 7 studies were included in the metaanalysis, remifentanil reduced the mean VAS scores at 1 hour by 25 mm compared with meperidine (95% CI, 20–29 mm). Compared with the sensitivity analysis of all 7 studies, the summary estimate of the 3-study analysis was unchanged, although the precision was reduced, as reflected by a wider CI.[24]

These studies showed that remifentanil reduced the mean VAS score more than meperidine. It is important to note that there is substantial clinical heterogeneity demonstrated in these studies with the drug regimens varying greatly.[24] Even though this systematic review included all studies involving laboring parturients, most studies excluded high-risk patients with obstetric complications, multiple gestation, and preterm labor. As a result, it is difficult to generalize the results to these populations. To better quantify the side effect profile and determine optimal dose regimens, large, well-conducted, randomized controlled trials that compare remifentanil with meperidine or other labor analgesics are recommended. The authors concluded that the optimal drug delivery doses and regimens remain to be determined.[24] No recommendations regarding dosing or implementation were provided.

In a 2008 review by Hill,[18] the use of remifentanil as an alternative to neuraxial anesthesia for labor is explored owing to "A growing number of women [who] either do not want or cannot have an epidural for labor." A total of 8 case reports and studies were included in this review. Evaluation of individual studies and statistical methods for comparing results are not included in this review.

Primary findings in this review related to the specific topic of interest indicate that remifentanil has been shown to provide effective analgesia, especially during the first stage of labor. The author states that remifentanil is currently the most suitable systemic opioid for obstetric use and, even though it has a rapid onset and offset, the timing cannot be matched to that of a single uterine contraction. Recommendations regarding dosing assert that the appropriate PCA dosing regimen is a 40-μg remifentanil bolus with a 2-minute lockout period. In the author's institution, remifentanil PCA is offered for routine use as a labor analgesic with dosing as stated. It is further recommended that parturients receiving PCA remifentanil should have one-to-one nursing care, availability of oxygen saturation monitoring, and oxygen supplementation if required.[18]

Van De Velde[25] (2005) concluded that "the analgesic efficiency of remifentanil for labor pain has been demonstrated and that it seems superior to other parenteral opioid alternatives." Van De Velde also states,

> We cannot at the moment recommend remifentanil for routine use in labor analgesia. However, with careful monitoring and skilled personnel present at all times in the labor and delivery ward, remifentanil is an option to treat certain patients in which more conventional options are contraindicated, as has been demonstrated by several other recent case reports.[25]

The recommendation indicates that a bolus between 0.2 and 0.5 μg/kg with a lockout period of 2 to 3 minutes and no background infusion seems to be a reasonable option.[25] Additional trials are recommended to establish maternal and neonatal safety of remifentanil use in this population.

A focused review of 9 studies that sought to summarize the efficacy of remifentanil as a labor analgesic was compiled and published in 2009 by Hinova and Fernando.[26] These investigators concluded that the analgesic effects and suitability of remifentanil for first-stage labor is well-supported. It was noted that the timing of dosing could not currently be matched to the cyclic nature of labor pain. The analysis of the studies included demonstrated that remifentanil produces clinically effective, but not complete, analgesia, with conversion rates to neuraxial analgesia of less than 10%.[26]

The investigators recommend an appropriate PCA dose regimen is a 40-μg remifentanil bolus with a 2-minute lockout. They strongly suggest that clinical guidelines be in place to ensure routine oxygen saturation monitoring, treatment of maternal desaturation with oxygen supplementation if needed, and one-to-one care using trained personnel.[26] Statistical evaluation of the individual studies and the methods used for comparing results are not included in this review. The authors state that more work is needed to establish the optimal drug administration regimen for remifentanil use in this population.

REMIFENTANIL COMPARED WITH OTHER PARENTERAL OPIOIDS

Three randomized controlled trials evaluated the efficacy of remifentanil compared with other narcotics administered parenterally for labor analgesia. In all 3 trials, remifentanil was compared with meperidine.[28–30] In addition to a comparison of remifentanil and meperidine, 1 trial also compared the efficacy of remifentanil and fentanyl.[29] Remifentanil was a more effective overall in all 3 studies.

A 2005 double-blind randomized controlled trial was conducted by Blair and colleagues[28] with the purpose of comparing the analgesic efficacy and safety of remifentanil with meperidine when both were administered using a PCA device. Forty parturients were selected randomly to receive either remifentanil 40 μg with a lockout of 2 minutes or meperidine 15 mg with a lockout of 10 minutes. An averaged dose (40 μg) rather than a calculated weight-based dose of remifentanil was chosen.

VAS scores for pain during the study and for overall pain were similar for both groups, with a mean score of 6.4 ± 1.5 cm for remifentanil and 6.9 ± 1.7 cm for meperidine. Overall satisfaction with analgesia in labor was higher for remifentanil and more women chose to continue using remifentanil up to and during delivery than chose to continue with meperidine. No recommendations were made by the authors regarding dosing or implementation in clinical practice.

A randomized, double-blind study by Douma and colleagues[29] was conducted to compare the analgesic efficacy of remifentanil with meperidine and fentanyl via PCA delivery. One hundred eighty parturients enrolled, and 159 completed the study. Fifty-two received remifentanil, 53 received meperidine, and 54 received fentanyl. The characteristics of the parturients did not differ statistically. Women allocated to the remifentanil group received a 40-μg loading dose, 40-μg boluses with a lockout of 2 minutes, and a maximum dose limit of 1200 μg/h. Those in the meperidine group received a 49.5-mg loading dose, 5-mg boluses with a 10-minute lockout, and maximum overall dose limit of 200 mg. Those in the fentanyl group received a 50-μg loading dose, boluses of 20 μg with a 5-minute lockout, and a maximum dose limit of 240 μg/h. P<.05 was considered statistically significant.

There was no difference in baseline pain scores between the groups, and in all groups the pain scores decreased significantly from baseline 1 hour after the start of treatment. Intergroup comparison showed that the decrease in pain scores after 1 hour was greater in the remifentanil group compared with the fentanyl and meperidine groups. After hours 2 and 3, the decrease in pain scores did not differ significantly between the 3 groups. In all groups, pain scores returned to pretreatment values within 3 hours after the initiation of treatment.[29]

The efficacy of meperidine, fentanyl, and remifentanil PCA for labor analgesia varied from mild to moderate in this study. Remifentanil PCA provided better analgesia than meperidine and fentanyl PCA during the first hour of treatment. The authors recommend the use of remifentanil only in the last phase of cervical dilation and with continuous monitoring. Further studies were recommended to determine the safety of remifentanil, especially with relation to its respiratory effects.[29]

Another double-blind randomized controlled trial evaluated was conducted by Evron and colleagues[30] in 2005. Eighty-eight healthy term parturients were enrolled in the study and were randomly assigned to receive either increasing doses of PCA remifentanil or an IV infusion of meperidine. For the 43 parturients randomized to receive remifentanil, each received a bolus of 20 μg as a starting dose, regardless of weight, with a 3-minute lockout interval. The dose was increased every 15 to 20 minutes by 5-μg increments, on patient request, to a maximum dose limit of 1500 μg/h. The 45 parturients who were randomized to the meperidine group received 75 mg of meperidine in 100 mL of normal saline over 30 minutes and in case of insufficient analgesia, another dose of 75 mg, followed by 50 mg when necessary, was administered, to a maximum dose of 200 mg of meperidine.

The authors concluded that PCA remifentanil use during labor and delivery was associated with improved VAS scores, higher patient satisfaction, and less need to cross over to epidural analgesia compared with IV meperidine. The use of remifentanil seemed to provide better analgesia than meperidine throughout labor and delivery and has minimal maternal or neonatal side effects. It was further stated that the findings in this study may justify the use of remifentanil as a systemic opioid in labor and delivery whenever there is a contraindication to neuraxial analgesia; however, a large study is still necessary to investigate the maternal and fetal side effects. Continuous monitoring of the oxygen saturation of the parturient is recommended to decrease the likelihood of maternal and neonatal hypoxemia.[30]

Although more and larger studies are justified, the evidence that currently exists supports the use of remifentanil. The efficacy of using remifentanil in managing parturient pain is clear, and should be considered as a mainstream medication of choice. Maternal and neonatal hypoxia are a risk for the use of any opioid analgesia (**Box 1**).

Remifentanil Compared with Neuraxial Anesthesia

The discussion thus far has identified contraindications neuraxial anesthesia, and a comparative analysis of medications used in parturient pain. The efficacy of

> **Box 1**
> **Important point**
>
> The efficacy of using remifentanil in managing parturient pain is clear, and should be considered as a mainstream medication of choice.

remifentanil is clearly supported. Now the focus is toward looking at the evidence that compares the use of remifentanil to neuraxial anesthesia.

There are 3 salient studies that looked at the use of remifentanil compared with neuraxial techniques, specifically epidural analgesia, which is considered the gold standard for management of labor pain.[5] In all 3 studies, neuraxial techniques were superior to remifentanil for the management of labor pain (**Box 2**).

Tveit and colleagues[31] conducted an randomized controlled trial, the stated objective of which was to compare the analgesic efficacy and side effects of remifentanil PCA with epidural analgesia during labor. Thirty-nine parturients were randomized to receive either remifentanil PCA or epidural anesthesia. The epidural contained ropivacaine 1 mg/mL and fentanyl 2 μg/mL; an initial bolus dose of 10 mL, followed by a 5 mL top-up after 5 minutes (total 15 mL) was given before the start of infusion at 10 mL/h. Thereafter, the midwife was allowed to adjust the infusion dose (5–15 mL/h) and give rescue doses of 5 mL if needed. The starting bolus of remifentanil was 0.15 μg/kg, and increases of 0.15 μg/kg were allowed every 15 minutes with no maximum limit. The PCA lockout time was 2 minutes, the bolus infusion speed was 2 mL/min (100 μg/min), and there was no background infusion. Owing to a technical problem with the infusion pumps after inclusion of 39 patients, the study was closed early, leaving the number of participants close to the estimation from the power calculation.

The mean baseline VAS pain scores were somewhat higher in the remifentanil group at 82 ± 13.3 versus 70 ± 16.2 mm for the epidural group, but the pain scores were reduced in both groups during the first hour of analgesia with the remifentanil group VAS of 38 ± 17.3 mm and the epidural group VAS 23 ± 30.2 mm ($P = .066$). Overall, there were no differences in pain reduction between parturients receiving remifentanil and epidural at the time points registered between 15 and 240 minutes. After 2 hours, pain scores in the remifentanil group tended to return toward baseline; thus, remifentanil seemed to produce less analgesia than epidural anesthesia in this phase of labor. The authors note that at the end of first and second stage, pain reduction was comparable between the groups, as was the maximal reduction in average pain score. The mean dose of ropivacaine was 33 mg (range, 5–84) and fentanyl dose of 67 μg (range, 10–168). Five patients received an extra bolus dose of 5 mL (rescue medication) because of unsatisfactory analgesia. A remifentanil mean dose of 0.40 μg/kg (range, 0.15–0.60) was reached after 1 hour. He maximum bolus dose during the study period was 0.70 μg/kg (range, 0.30–1.05). The mean doses at the end of the first and second stages were 0.65 and 0.38 μg/kg (ranges of 0.30–1.05 and 0.15–0.90), respectively.[31]

The authors concluded that both treatments provided good analgesia, but that there were higher pain scores in the remifentanil group. Pain reduction at the end of first and during second stage and maximum pain reduction were similar. Based on current

> **Box 2**
> **Important point**
>
> In all 3 studies, neuraxial techniques were superior to remifentanil for the management of labor pain.

knowledge, the authors recommend the maximum remifentanil dose should not exceed 0.7 μg/kg and that remifentanil PCA be used as a stepwise bolus dose regimen, with dose steps of 0.15 μg/kg and a 2-minute lockout time. Large-scale, randomized, controlled trials are recommended to assess dosing regimens, analgesic efficacy, and side effects.[31]

A 2011 study by Ismail and Hassanin[32] sought to determine the difference in duration of labor, the mode of delivery, average VAS pain scores, maternal overall satisfaction with analgesia, side effects, and neonatal outcomes in nulliparous women who received early labor analgesia with either epidural, PCA with remifentanil, or combined spinal–epidural (CSE) techniques. The study included 1140 healthy parturients who were randomized to receive either epidural analgesia (n = 380), PCA remifentanil (n = 380), or CSE analgesia (n = 380). The primary outcome measured was the rate of cesarean delivery. In the epidural group, an 8-mL dose of 0.125% levobupivacaine with 2 μg/mL fentanyl was administered through the epidural catheter and a continuous infusion of 8 mL/h of 0.125% levobupivacaine and 2 μg/mL fentanyl was initiated. Further boluses of 5 to 10 mL of 0.125% levobupivacaine were given upon request. In the CSE group, a needle-through-needle technique was performed with 2 mg levobupivacaine and 15 μg fentanyl (total volume of 2 mL) injected intrathecally with the epidural catheter inserted and connected to the same continuous infusion used in the epidural group. In the remifentanil group, the PCA device was set to deliver 0.1 μg/kg of remifentanil diluted with saline and given as a solution of 25 μg/mL as a bolus infused over a period of 1 minute, with a lockout time of 1 minute. During the study, the PCA bolus was increased following a dose escalation scheme (0.1–0.2–0.3–0.5–0.7–0.9 μg/kg) after every second contraction until the parturient answered "no" to the question whether she would like to get more efficient pain relief or until a maximum dose of 0.9 μg/kg was achieved.[32]

No differences were observed among the 3 groups with regard to average VAS score at analgesia request (epidural group, 64.5 ± 12.84 mm; remifentanil group, 66.4 ± 11.50 mm; CSE group, 65.8 ± 12.10 mm; P = .089). The CSE group showed a score of 22.56 ± 7.57 mm versus 34.3 ± 9.8 mm for remifentanil and 35.6 ± 10.2 mm for epidural (P = .000). The authors concluded in terms of labor duration, average VAS pain scores, and maternal overall satisfaction score with analgesia, CSE analgesia is superior to that provided by epidural analgesia or PCA with remifentanil for pain relief. There were no differences in the mode of delivery, side effects, or neonatal outcomes between the 3 techniques.[32] Other than the method used within the study, no further recommendations regarding remifentanil PCA dosing or implementation were provided.

A randomized clinical trial that compared remifentanil and neuraxial techniques was published by Stocki and colleagues[33] in 2014. The primary objective was to demonstrate noninferiority of remifentanil labor analgesia compared with epidural analgesia in laboring women. Thirty-nine parturients participated with random allocation of 19 in the remifentanil group and 20 in the epidural group. Remifentanil was given as a bolus dose and titrated to effect from 20 μg up to a maximum of 60 μg as required with an initial lockout interval of 2 minutes and no background infusion. The PCA bolus/lockout interval was titrated to an endpoint of either patient comfort or a maximal bolus dose of 60 μg/minimal lockout interval of 1 minute. For the epidural group, an incremental initial loading dose of 15 mL of 0.1% bupivacaine with 50 μg fentanyl was administered followed by patient-controlled epidural analgesia infusion of 0.1% bupivacaine with fentanyl 2 μg/mL. A basal infusion of 5 mL/h, with patient-controlled bolus of 10 mL and a 20-minute lockout was initiated. Additional epidural bolus doses (either 0.1% bupivacaine 10 mL during the first stage of labor or 1% lidocaine 8 mL during the second stage of labor) were administered to treat breakthrough pain.[33]

In this study, maternal pain was assessed using an 11-point verbal numerical rating scale (NRS) of 0 [no pain] to 10 [the worst pain imaginable]. There was no difference found between baseline NRS pain scores in the 2 groups. Both remifentanil and epidural analgesia resulted in a significant decrease from baseline NRS scores over time. It was observed that scores were significantly lower at 30 minutes in both groups with change for remifentanil of -4.7 ± 0.6 and -7.2 ± 0.6 for epidural ($P<.0001$). Although both modalities are effective at reducing NRS pain scores, remifentanil is inferior to epidural with regard to the magnitude of the pain score reduction at all time points. Pain scores were higher at all time points than an expected -1.5-unit difference in NRS scores. The authors state that, "a 'safe' dose or duration of administration of remifentanil cannot be recommended based on the results presented in this study."[33] They concluded that remifentanil administration for labor requires appropriate monitoring to detect and alert for maternal apnea and, although remifentanil analgesia is inferior to epidural analgesia, it may provide a satisfactory alternative when epidural analgesia is not desired or permitted. It is further stated that future studies should consider remifentanil use in the obstetric population with particular focus on respiratory monitoring and manpower requirements for implementation (**Box 3**).[33]

Methods of Delivery: An Important Consideration

Three trials specifically address the delivery of remifentanil when used as the primary analgesic for the management of labor pain. The methods investigated are PCA with a background infusion, PCA without a background infusion, and a continuous remifentanil infusion without any patient control.

Balki and colleagues[34] conducted a prospective randomized controlled trial in 2007 to compare the efficacy of 2 regimens of remifentanil PCA implemented for labor analgesia to determine an optimal dosing regimen. Twenty parturients were randomized into 2 groups. Remifentanil was administered as a 50 μg/mL solution with all patients initially receiving a standard regimen of an infusion of 0.025 μg/kg/min and a PCA bolus of 0.25 μg/kg with a 2-minute lockout and 4-hour limit of 3 mg. As labor progressed and the patients required additional analgesia, they received higher doses of either the infusion or the PCA boluses, depending on the group to which they had been randomly assigned.

In the variable infusion, fixed bolus group, the infusion rate was increased stepwise from 0.025 to 0.05 μg/kg/min, 0.075 μg/kg/min, and 0.1 μg/kg/min, and the bolus of 0.25 μg/kg remained unchanged. In the variable bolus, fixed infusion group, the bolus dose was increased stepwise from 0.25 to 0.5 μg/kg, 0.75 μg/kg, and 1 μg/kg, and the infusion rate of 0.025 μg/kg/min was kept constant. Each step was maintained for at least 15 minutes before progressing to the subsequent one.

The mean pain and patient satisfaction scores, and cumulative doses of remifentanil, were similar in the 2 groups. The overall difference in pain scores between the groups were not significant. The variable infusion, fixed bolus group had a mean

---

Box 3
Important point

In the randomized clinical trial, it was found that, although remifentanil analgesia is inferior to epidural analgesia, it may provide a satisfactory alternative when epidural analgesia is not desired or permitted.

pain score of 6.09 ± 0.49 and the variable bolus, fixed infusion group had a score of 5.51 ± 0.46 (P = .40) According to the authors, this pilot study suggests that remifentanil PCA is efficacious for labor analgesia. They recommend delivery of remifentanil as a bolus of 0.25 μg/kg with a 2-minute lockout and continuous background infusion of 0.025 to 0.1 μg/kg/min. Close monitoring of respiratory status and vitals was mandated and further trials were recommended.[34]

A 2013 prospective, randomized, double-blinded, randomized, controlled trial conducted by Shen and colleagues[35] aimed to compare the effects of remifentanil for labor analgesia given by either PCA or continuous infusion. Sixty parturients were randomized to be in either the PCA group, to whom remifentanil was administered using increasing stepwise boluses from 0.1 to 0.4 μg/kg in 0.1-μg/kg increments with a 2-minute lockout, or in the continuous infusion group, which used rates from 0.05 to 0.2 μg/kg/min with incremental increases of 0.05 μg/kg/min given on request.

The demographic variables, patient characteristics, remifentanil concentrations, and umbilical cord blood gases analysis were compared. The maternal and neonatal adverse reactions and fetal heart rate tracings were analyzed.[35] The 2 groups were similar regarding patient characteristics. Pain scores were significantly lower at 30, 60, and 90 minutes in the PCA group and the pain relief scores were significantly higher at 60, 90, 120 minutes compared with those in the infusion group. Women reported lowest pain scores of 3 (range, 2–5) for PCA and 4 (range, 3–7) for continuous infusion at 60 minutes after the beginning of analgesia. The total remifentanil consumption during PCA administration was lower than continuous infusion with PCA group consumption of 1.34 mg (range, 0.89–1.69) versus 1.49 mg (range, 1.12–1.70) for the continuous infusion group (P = .011). According to the authors, the results suggest that remifentanil administered with an incremental PCA bolus is a preferable alternative to continuous infusion because it provides better pain relief, but with similar maternal side effects and placental transfer. They further state that continuous monitoring of SPO_2 and oxygen supplementation during IV remifentanil analgesia is essential.[35]

A randomized study by Balcioglu and colleagues[36] conducted in 2007 sought to assess and compare the efficiency and safety of the PCA use of remifentanil combined with 2 different supplementary background infusions. Sixty subjects were divided into 2 groups. Both groups received the same fixed loading and demand remifentanil doses of 20 and 15 μg, respectively, with a 5-minute lockout between bolus doses. One group then received a background infusion of 0.1 μg/kg/min and the other a background infusion at 0.15 μg/kg/min. Meperidine was available in addition to the remifentanil if pain was not controlled. All the data were collected by the same anesthesiologist and expressed as mean ± standard deviation or median (range). The differences in hemodynamic parameters, VAS pain scores, and sedation scores were statistically compared.

Demographic data and labor characteristics of the 2 groups were statistically comparable and mean VAS values of the groups were similar at baseline. After PCA administration of remifentanil, the mean pain score significantly decreased at the 5-minute measurement and remained at low levels (VAS < 2) in both groups (P<.05). The mean pain score of the group receiving the 0.15 μg/kg/min infusion was significantly lower than that of the group receiving 0.10 μg/kg/min throughout labor and delivery (P<.05). No additional drug was needed for pain relief. There were no differences between the total remifentanil consumption levels of the groups with 2.4 ± 0.7 mg for the 0.1 μg/kg/min group versus 2.6 ± 0.4 mg for the 0.15 μg/kg/min group. Parturients in the group with the lower background infusion asked for more bolus than the other group. The authors concluded that, for effective analgesia, PCA of remifentanil with a 15-µg demand dose and 0.15-µg/kg/min background infusion is a better choice than a 0.10-µg/kg/min infusion. They recommend that implementation occur with careful maternal and fetal monitoring.[36]

DOSING AND TIMING

Two studies address the subjects of the dosing and timing of remifentanil for labor analgesia. Neither study produced any particular significant recommendations related to either the timing or dosing regimen and are therefore only briefly addressed and not fully detailed.

One study addressing this topic was a prospective, randomized, single-blind, crossover conducted by Jost and colleagues[37] to investigate differences in the analgesic efficiency, safety, and drug consumption between a modified bolus delivery regimen the authors developed and a "classical" regimen. Both regimens included continuous background infusion with the rate of around 0.010 µg/kg/min and PCA boluses upon request. The classical regimen was 20-µg bolus increased upon the request of a parturient up to 30 µg after 20 minutes, 35 µg after 1 hour, and 45 µg after 2 hours, and 55 µg after 3 hours with a bolus infusion rate of 1.2 µg/s. The modified regimen was based on the duration of time the patient depressed the delivery button on the PCA. The regimen had a starting bolus infusion rate of 3 µg/s with a stepwise decrease of 20% of the initial rate every 6 seconds and terminating bolus delivery by either releasing the PCA button or reaching the maximum bolus dose of 60 µg.

No serious side effects or complications were observed in the study. There were no differences in observed parameters except for slightly lower blood pressure with the modified regimen. Pain estimates were lower in women starting with the modified regimen with average estimated VAS scores of 54 mm for the classical regimen and 45 mm for the modified regimen ($P = .005$). There were fewer requests for analgesia within the lockout period (31 vs 69; $P = .041$) and fewer bolus adjustments (0 vs 25; $P<.001$) with the modified regimen. The authors note several limitations within this study and state they believe that the benefits of the modified regimen outlined herein were not fully demonstrated in this study.[37] No practical dosing or timing information was presented.

Another study focused on the dosing and timing of remifentanil for labor analgesia and was conducted by Volmanen and colleagues[38] in 2011. In this study, it was hypothesized that the timing of the bolus in the contraction cycle could have importance and administering a remifentanil bolus during contraction pause would improve analgesia in early labor. Fifty parturients participated in this double-blind crossover study. Remifentanil dose of 0.4 µg/kg with a 1-minute infusion time was used during 2 study periods lasting 6 to 8 contractions. Remifentanil and saline syringes were attached to 2 PCA devices, one of which administered the bolus immediately after a trigger and the other targeted to start 140 seconds before the next contraction. Group 1 (n = 25) received a bolus immediately after the PCA signal during the first period and after a delay during the latter period, whereas group 2 (n = 25) received the dosing regimens in reverse order. A lockout period of 1 minute was used.

Statistical analysis showed that there was no difference in the duration of the study periods or the average contraction interval between the 2 dosing regimens. When the study periods were analyzed separately by comparing the groups as in parallel studies, there was no difference in the pain scores or the variables related to the analgesic effect. When the 2 groups were analyzed together, the mean of the pain scores during contractions was 3.3 during the first study period and 5.3 during the second

(P<.001). Remifentanil consumed during the first period was 0.067 µg/kg/min and 0.077 µg/kg/min during the second (P<.007). Interestingly, the first study period (immediate dosing) was preferred by both groups. The authors state that the main finding of this study was that the timing of the administration of a remifentanil bolus during the uterine contraction cycle has no significance related to the timing in which a 1-utemin PCA bolus is given. No further recommendations regarding timing or implementation were made.[38]

PUTTING THIS ALL TOGETHER

Each of these studies were analyzed for the remifentanil dosing regimen and implementation method used. The doses, implementation methods, and recommendations found in each study are presented in **Table 2**. If a recommended dose or method of implementation was not given specifically, the dose and method used in conduction of the study was used as the recommended dose.

The overall number of studies specifically investigating the use of remifentanil in parturients are few and most look at only a small fraction of the overall parturient population. Among the specific population of interest—parturients for whom neuraxial anesthesia is not an option—the body of literature contained only a few case studies and these lacked the scientific rigor required to be included in evaluation of this topic. The literature included in this review demonstrated clinical heterogeneity; different study protocols with respect to implementation methods, dosing, timing, rate of administration, lockout intervals, and comparative drugs make it difficult to conduct a comparison. Participants in the included studies were quite homogeneous in nature, with most being healthy American Society of Anesthesiologists physical status 1 or 2 patients who met relatively strict inclusion criteria. This is a very specific body of literature related to the efficacious and safe use of remifentanil as a labor analgesic.

THE IMPORTANCE OF SAFETY

An issue that was presented in a majority of the studies is that of safety related to remifentanil use in this application. Frequently, assessed parameters that were often a secondary focus of the studies included maternal blood pressure, SPO_2, $ETCO_2$, respiratory rate, and level of sedation. In addition, fetal/neonatal assessment often included fetal heart rate, umbilical cord pH, and 1- and 5-minute Apgar scores as a measure of assessing adverse response to remifentanil use for labor analgesia. On the maternal side of the safety discussion, most literature suggested that close monitoring of SPO_2, respiratory rate, and level of sedation be undertaken with the use of remifentanil.

In addition to monitoring, the use of supplemental oxygen was also frequently recommended and was implemented in many of the studies. Another frequent recommendation that many authors made was the necessity of having individual nursing care when remifentanil is used in the parturient.[18,26,29–31] It is also important to note that many studies investigating the feasibility of remifentanil reported a low number of adverse maternal and fetal events. This low number of adverse events may, therefore, cause an overestimation of the safety of remifentanil use in labor.[23]

ETHICAL CONSIDERATIONS

The ethical issues surrounding the use of remifentanil for labor analgesia require consideration before use in clinical practice. The evidence supports the use of remifentanil in the parturient as an acceptable practice. The evidence also supports that

Table 2
Summary of remifentanil dosing regiment and implementation method used

Author	Implementation Method	Remifentanil Dose Used	Recommendation
Schnabel et al,[23] 2012	N/A	N/A	No recommendation.
Leong et al,[24] 2011	N/A	N/A	No recommendation.
Hill,[18] 2008	N/A	N/A	40 μg remifentanil bolus, 2-min lockout.
Van De Velde,[25] 2005	N/A	N/A	0.2–0.5 μg/kg bolus, 2- to 3-min lockout, no background infusion.
Hinova and Fernando,[26] 2009	N/A	N/A	40 μg bolus, 2-min lockout.
Blair et al,[28] 2005	Fixed PCA bolus	40-μg bolus, 2-min lockout.	40-μg bolus, 2-min lockout.
Douma et al,[29] 2010	Fixed PCA bolus + loading dose	40-μg loading dose, 40-μg per bolus, 2-min lockout.	40-μg loading dose, 40 μg per bolus, 2-min lockout.
Evron et al,[30] 2005	Stepwise ↑ PCA bolus	20-μg starting dose, 3 min lockout, ↑ in 5-μg increments every 15–20 min on request.	20-μg starting dose, 3 min lockout, ↑ in 5-μg increments every 15–20 min on request.
Tveit et al,[31] 2012	Stepwise ↑ PCA bolus	Starting bolus 0.15 μg/kg, 0.15 μg/kg ↑ every 15 min on request.	PCA as a stepwise bolus dose regimen, dose steps of 0.15 μg/kg, 2-min lockout, maximum dose 0.7 μg/kg.
Ismail and Hassanin,[32] 2012	Stepwise ↑ PCA bolus	0.1 μg/kg bolus infused over 1 min, 1 min lockout, bolus ↑ 0.1 μg/kg after every second contraction until satisfaction stated with current dose or maximum dose of 0.9 μg/kg.	0.1 μg/kg bolus, 1 min lockout, bolus ↑ 0.1 μg/kg until satisfied or maximum dose of 0.9 μg/kg.
Stocki et al,[33] 2014	Stepwise ↑ PCA bolus	20-μg bolus ↑ to 60 μg maximum as required, 2-min initial lockout, no background infusion. Bolus dose and lockout interval titrated to patient comfort or a maximum bolus 60 μg and 1-min lockout.	20-μg bolus ↑ as required, 2-min initial lockout. Bolus dose and lockout interval titrated to patient comfort or a maximum bolus 60 μg and 1-min lockout. No background infusion.

(continued on next page)

Table 2
(continued)

Author	Implementation Method	Remifentanil Dose Used	Recommendation
Balki et al,[34] 2007	Stepwise ↑ PCA bolus or infusion rate	Infusion ↑ from 0.025 µg/kg/min in 0.025-µg increments up to 0.1 µg/kg/min, bolus of 0.25 µg/kg unchanged. Bolus ↑ from 0.25 µg/kg in 0.25-µg increments up to 1 µg/kg, infusion rate of 0.025 µg/kg/min unchanged.	0.25-µg/kg bolus, 2- min lockout, background infusion 0.025–0.1 µg/kg/min.
Shen et al,[35] 2013	Stepwise ↑ PCA bolus or infusion rate	0.1-µg/kg bolus, 2-min lockout, ↑ in 0.1-µg/kg increments to 0.4 µg/kg maximum. Continuous infusion 0.05 µg/kg/min, ↑ by 0.05-µg/kg/min increments on request, maximum 0.2 µg/kg/min.	0.1-µg/kg bolus, 2-min lockout, ↑ in 0.1-µg/kg increments to 0.4 µg/kg maximum. No background infusion.
Balcioglu et al,[36] 2007	Fixed PCA bolus + loading dose + background infusion	20-µg loading dose, 15-µg bolus, 5 min lockout. Background infusion of either 0.1 or 0.15 µg/kg/min.	15-µg bolus, 5-min lockout, 0.15-µg/kg/min background infusion.
Jost et al,[37] 2013	Stepwise ↑ PCA bolus + continuous infusion	Classic = infusion 0.010 µg/kg/min + 20-µg boluses on request, ↑ to 30 µg after 20 min, 35 µg after 1 h, 45 µg after 2 h, and 55 µg after 3 h. Modified based on time button pressed. Starting rate 3 µg/s with a stepwise ↓ 20% of initial rate every 6 s, terminate at button release or 60 µg maximum dose.	
Volmanen et al,[38] 2011	Fixed PCA bolus	0.4-µg/kg bolus, 1-min infusion time, 1-min lockout. Traditional: bolus immediately. Other: bolus 140 s before next contraction	0.4-µg/kg bolus, 1-min infusion time, 1-min lockout.

Abbreviations: N/A, not applicable; PCA, patent-controlled analgesia.

the use of this regimen can potentially expand access to pain relief during labor for those who may otherwise be excluded. The relief of pain is a basic human right and as such should not be denied.[3] Remifentanil use meets this need for the relief of pain during labor. The expansion of access and the relief of pain are certainly positive attributes of the use of remifentanil in the parturient.

There are, however, other aspects of ethical concern that each practitioner who accepts the responsibility of providing for a patient requiring or desiring remifentanil as a labor analgesic must take into consideration. It is important to emphasize that every clinical situation in which remifentanil may be used requires a thorough evaluation by the practitioner of not only applicable clinical data, but also of the patient and their individual needs during the birthing process.

Not only must the patient be considered in this discussion, but also the unborn child who is wholly dependent on the physiologic homeostasis provided by the mother. The use of remifentanil as a labor analgesic has proven to be both safe and effective when implemented properly. Several studies have examined the side effects of remifentanil use during the first and second stages of labor and the occurrence of serious adverse events or poor neonatal outcomes is rare.[18,28–36] This is not to say that the use of remifentanil is totally without risk. Maternal adverse events, such as apnea and hypoxia, do occur and there are case reports of more serious events, such as cardiac arrest, that have occurred with the use of remifentanil as a labor analgesic.[39,40]

Another major consideration when contemplating the use of remifentanil in this application is that of the risks versus the benefits. The risks and benefits of remifentanil use have been discussed. The risk for an adverse event is increased by several factors, including unfamiliarity with the remifentanil protocol, inadequate staff education, inability to provide individual nursing care, and unrealistic expectations by patients and staff.

The benefits of implementation may be either physical or nonphysical in nature. For example, a patient with thrombocytopenia owing to preeclampsia and may be physically unable to tolerate any further increases in blood pressure caused by the pain of labor without becoming eclamptic; in this situation, the use of remifentanil has the potential keep the pain manageable and blood pressure out of the eclamptic range. A benefit that is nonphysical in nature may be that of a sense of self-control over the analgesia being administered.[25] By giving the parturient the control offered by a PCA, she is able to determine the level of analgesia that is appropriate based on her needs and desires. Again, this assessment of risks and benefits requires that the clinician thoroughly evaluate clinically relevant information as well as the individual needs and desires of the patient and then tailor the anesthetic plan accordingly.

A final thought regarding the ethical considerations of remifentanil use in the parturient is centered on the costs associated with not only the drug, but also with implementation. This potent, short-acting narcotic is more expensive when compared with less efficacious narcotics or local anesthetics traditionally used in the management of labor pain.[41,42] In addition to the cost of the drug, safe implementation requires additional equipment such as $ETCO_2$ monitoring and additional staff to provide individual nursing care. The costs vary by locale, but there may be a substantial increase in costs to the facility with the implementation of this regimen. These increases in the cost of caring for 1 patient may deplete resources available for other patients and in turn, negatively affect the care that they receive owing to financial constraints. Cost savings may be realized by reducing vital precautions but, in so doing, may lead to catastrophic outcomes.[43]

One must consider if the risks of remifentanil use are commensurate to the benefits and, if so, whether the benefits then justify the cost. The value of the alleviating pain —whether it is physical or mental—indicates that each provider must answer these questions that arise regarding the use of remifentanil by using his or her own clinical knowledge, personal and professional beliefs, and the individual needs and desires of patients before coming to a decision based on that information.

EVIDENCE-BASED RECOMMENDATION

Based on a thorough review of literature on the subject of remifentanil use in the parturient for whom neuraxial anesthesia is not an option, the use of remifentanil as a labor analgesic is an acceptable practice. The use of remifentanil is considered off-label for obstetric use and there is currently no consensus on the optimal dosing regimen.[17,18] Large-scale studies with rigorous guidelines and protocols need to be conducted to procure further evidence regarding the optimal use of remifentanil in the parturient. These recommendations would ideally include implementation information and order guidelines for the anesthetist, implementation and usage guidelines for nursing staff, and educational information for patients.

Table 3 displays the recommendations for anesthesia providers that desire to use remifentanil for labor analgesia in the parturient. A PCA bolus of 40 μg with a 2-minute lockout and no background infusion is recommended. Supplemental oxygen should be used in conjunction with continuous monitoring of SPO_2, $ETCO_2$, and cardiotocograph readings. Vital signs (blood pressure, heart rate, respiratory rate, SPO_2, $ETCO_2$, level of consciousness, and pain) should be documented on a Remifentanil PCA flow sheet every 5 minutes for the first 30 minutes after initiating PCA and then every 15 minutes for the duration of remifentanil use. Individual nursing care should be provided and the nurse should have advanced cardiovascular life support certification.

Table 3 Putting it all together	
Mixture	Remifentanil 2 mg diluted in 50 mL normal saline (40 μg/mL)
Delivery method	PCA
Dosing	40-μg bolus 2-min lockout
Implementation	Dedicated IV site for remifentanil with carrier fluid running at 100 mL/h O_2 via nasal cannula @ 2-3 L/min

Monitoring/documentation	Continuous SPO_2 monitoring with audible alarm for ≤93%
	Continuous $ETCO_2$ monitoring with audible alarms for ≥55 mm Hg
	Continuous cardiotocograph monitoring
	Vitals (BP, HR, RR, SPO_2, $ETCO_2$, LOC, pain)
	   Every 5 min for the first 30 min after initiating PCA
	   Then every 15 min for the duration of remifentanil use
	All times and vitals documented on remifentanil flow sheet
	Reconciliation per facility protocol of remifentanil use and waste

Staffing	1:1 nursing care with ACLS trained provider Supervising anesthetist in-house and immediately available
Other	Concomitant use of other opioid analgesics is not recommended

Abbreviations: ACLS, advanced cardiac life support; BP, blood pressure; HR, heart rate; IV, intravenous; LOC, level of consciousness; PCA, patent-controlled analgesia; RR, respiratory rate.

It is further recommended that the supervising anesthetist be in house and immediately available for the entire duration of remifentanil use. Concomitant use of other opioid analgesics is not recommended. These recommendations are an amalgamation of evidence gleaned from the studies analyzed and should not be considered absolute. CRNAs must take into account their own clinical knowledge as well as individual patient needs and desires before implementing remifentanil in the parturient.

ACKNOWLEDGMENTS

The author would to acknowledge the kind assistance Dr. Rachel Brown, CRNA, and Michael Vollman, PhD, RN, in the preparation of this article.

REFERENCES

1. Olufolabi AJ, Booth JV, Wakeling HG, et al. A preliminary investigation of remifentanil as a labor analgesic. Anesth Analg 2000;91(3):606–8.
2. Pain definitions. IASP website. http://www.iasp-pain.org/Content/NavigationMenu/GeneralResourceLinks/PainDefinitions/default.htm. Accessed December 1, 2013.
3. Brennan F, Carr D, Cousins M. Pain management: a fundamental human right. Anesth Analg 2007;105(1):205–21.
4. Melzack R. The myth of painless childbirth (the John J. Bonica lecture). Pain 1984;19(4):321–37.
5. Chestnut DH. Obstetric anesthesia, principles and practice. Philadelphia: Elsevier Health Sciences; 2004.
6. Begley CE, Lairson DR, Morgan RO, et al. Evaluating the healthcare system: effectiveness, efficiency, and equity. 4th edition. Chicago: Health Administration Press; 2013.
7. Lehmann KA. Recent developments in patient-controlled analgesia. J Pain Symptom Manage 2005;29(5 Suppl):S72–89.
8. Hodnett ED. Pain and women's satisfaction with the experience of childbirth: a systematic review. Am J Obstet Gynecol 2002;186(5 Suppl Nature):S160–72.
9. Dulisse B, Cromwell J. No harm found when nurse anesthetists work without supervision by physicians. Health Aff 2010;29:1469–75.
10. Nagelhout J, Plaus K. Nurse anesthesia. St Louis (MO): Saunders/Elsevier; 2010.
11. Miller RD. Miller's anesthesia. 5th edition. Philadelphia: Churchill Livingstone/Elsevier; 2010. c2010.
12. Mikhail M, Murray MJ. Clinical anesthesiology. New York: McGraw-Hill Medical; 2005.
13. Brunton L, Blumenthal D, Buxton I, et al. Goodman and Gilman's manual of pharmacology and therapeutics. New York: McGraw Hill Professional; 2007.
14. Stoelting RK, Hillier SC. Pharmacology and physiology in anesthetic practice. Philadelphia: Lippincott Williams & Wilkins; 2012.
15. Beers R, Camporesi E. Remifentanil update: clinical science and utility. CNS Drugs 2004;18(15):1085–104.
16. Glass PS, Hardman D, Kamiyama Y, et al. Preliminary pharmacokinetics and pharmacodynamics of an ultra-short-acting opioid: remifentanil (GI87084B). Anesth Analg 1993;77(5):1031–40.
17. Sneyd JR. Recent advances in intravenous anaesthesia. Br J Anaesth 2004; 93(5):725–36.
18. Hill D. The use of remifentanil in obstetrics. Anesthesiol Clin 2008;26(1):169–82, viii.
19. Horlocker TT, Wedel DJ, Rowlingson JC, et al. Regional anesthesia in the patient receiving antithrombotic or thrombolytic therapy: American Society of Regional

Anesthesia and Pain Medicine evidence-based guidelines (third edition). Reg Anesth Pain Med 2010;35(1):64–101.

20. Daley MD, Rolbin SH, Hew EM, et al. Epidural anesthesia for obstetrics after spinal surgery. Reg Anesth 1990;15(6):280–4.

21. Smith PS, Wilson RC, Robinson AP, et al. Regional blockade for delivery in women with scoliosis or previous spinal surgery. Int J Obstet Anesth 2003;12(1):17–22.

22. Cousins MJ, Bridenbaugh PO, Carr DB, et al. Cousins and Bridenbaugh's neural blockade in clinical anesthesia and pain medicine. Philadelphia: Lippincott Williams & Wilkins; 2009.

23. Schnabel A, Hahn N, Broscheit J, et al. Remifentanil for labour analgesia: a meta-analysis of randomised controlled trials. Eur J Anaesthesiol 2012;29(4): 177–85.

24. Leong WL, Sng BL, Sia AT. A comparison between remifentanil and meperidine for labor analgesia: a systematic review. Anesth Analg 2011;113(4):818–25.

25. Van de Velde M. Remifentanil for obstetric analgesia and anesthesia: a review of the literature. Acta Anaesthesiol Belg 2005;56(1):45–9.

26. Hinova A, Fernando R. Systemic remifentanil for labor analgesia. Anesth Analg 2009;109(6):1925–9.

27. Ullman R, Smith LA, Burns E, et al. Parenteral opioids for maternal pain relief in labour. Cochrane Database Syst Rev 2010;(9):CD007396.

28. Blair JM, Dobson GT, Hill DA, et al. Patient controlled analgesia for labour: a comparison of remifentanil with pethidine. Anaesthesia 2005;60(1):22–7.

29. Douma MR, Verwey RA, Kam-endtz CE, et al. Obstetric analgesia: a comparison of patient-controlled meperidine, remifentanil, and fentanyl in labour. Br J Anaesth 2010;104(2):209–15.

30. Evron S, Glezerman M, Sadan O, et al. Remifentanil: a novel systemic analgesic for labor pain. Anesth Analg 2005;100(1):233–8.

31. Tveit TO, Seiler S, Halvorsen A, et al. Labour analgesia: a randomised, controlled trial comparing intravenous remifentanil and epidural analgesia with ropivacaine and fentanyl. Eur J Anaesthesiol 2012;29(3):129–36.

32. Ismail MT, Hassanin MZ. Neuraxial analgesia versus intravenous remifentanil for pain relief in early labor in nulliparous women. Arch Gynecol Obstet 2012;286(6): 1375–81.

33. Stocki D, Matot I, Einav S, et al. A randomized controlled trial of the efficacy and respiratory effects of patient-controlled intravenous remifentanil analgesia and patient-controlled epidural analgesia in laboring women. Anesth Analg 2014; 118(3):589–97.

34. Balki M, Kasodekar S, Dhumne S, et al. Remifentanil patient-controlled analgesia for labour: optimizing drug delivery regimens. Can J Anaesth 2007;54(8):626–33.

35. Shen MK, Wu ZF, Zhu AB, et al. Remifentanil for labour analgesia: a double-blinded, randomised controlled trial of maternal and neonatal effects of patient-controlled analgesia versus continuous infusion. Anaesthesia 2013; 68(3):236–44.

36. Balcioglu O, Akin S, Demir S, et al. Patient-controlled intravenous analgesia with remifentanil in nulliparous subjects in labor. Expert Opin Pharmacother 2007; 8(18):3089–96.

37. Jost A, Ban B, Kamenik M. Modified patient-controlled remifentanil bolus delivery regimen for labour pain. Anaesthesia 2013;68(3):245–52.

38. Volmanen PV, Akural EI, Raudaskoski T, et al. Timing of intravenous patient-controlled remifentanil bolus during early labour. Acta Anaesthesiol Scand 2011;55(4):486–94.

39. Marr R, Hyams J, Bythell V. Cardiac arrest in an obstetric patient using remifentanil patient-controlled analgesia. Anaesthesia 2013;68(3):283–7.
40. Bonner JC, Mcclymont W. Respiratory arrest in an obstetric patient using remifentanil patient-controlled analgesia. Anaesthesia 2012;67(5):538–40.
41. Remifentanil cost. ACE Surgical Supply Co., Inc. Available at: http://www.acesurgical.com/ultiva-remifentanil-powder-1mg-10x3ml.html. Accessed August 18, 2014.
42. Meperidine cost. ACE Surgical Supply Co., Inc. Available at: http://www.acesurgical.com/demerol-100mg-ml-20ml-vial.html. Accessed August 18, 2014.
43. Kranke P, Girard T, Lavand'homme P, et al. Must we press on until a young mother dies? Remifentanil patient controlled analgesia in labour may not be suited as a "poor man's epidural". BMC Pregnancy Childbirth 2013;13:139.

Using Complementary and Alternative Medicine to Treat Pain and Agitation in Dementia

A Review of Randomized Controlled Trials from Long-Term Care with Potential Use in Critical Care

Alison R. Anderson, MSN, NP-C, ANP-BC[a],*, Jie Deng, PhD, RN, OCN[a], Robert S. Anthony, BS[a], Sebastian A. Atalla, BS[a], Todd B. Monroe, PhD, RN-BC, FNAP, FGSA[a,b]

KEYWORDS

- Pain • Agitation • Dementia • CAM • Aromatherapy • Essential oil • Massage
- Touch

KEY POINTS

- Behavioral and psychological symptoms of dementia, such as agitation, may indicate or be exacerbated by, pain.
- Pain in dementia is undertreated and there is a need for noninvasive, safe, and gentle pain management options.
- Complementary and alternative medicine therapies are becoming more popular and widely used with positive attitudes toward and satisfaction with use, and should be continued when indicated.
- Although aromatherapy did not show efficacy in dementia, it was found to be safe and promotes reduced stress in nurses and staff working in critical care.
- Massage, touch, and human interaction and presence have demonstrated efficacy in reducing stress, agitation, and pain in individuals with dementia and can be used in critical care.

Disclosure Statement: The authors have nothing to disclose.
This work was supported by the John A. Hartford Foundation, Mayday Fund, Vanderbilt Office of Clinical and Translational Scientist Development, Vanderbilt Clinical and Translational Research Scholars Program, and the National Institutes of Health National Institute on Aging (grants number K23 AG046379-01A1, number R21 AG045735-01A1, and R21 AG045735-01A1). The contents are solely the responsibility of the authors and do not necessarily represent the official views of these institutions.
[a] Vanderbilt University School of Nursing, Vanderbilt University, 461 21st Avenue South, Nashville, TN 37240, USA; [b] Department of Psychiatry and Behavioral Health, Vanderbilt University School of Medicine, Vanderbilt University, 461 21st Avenue South, Nashville, TN 37240, USA
* Corresponding author.
E-mail address: alison.r.anderson@vanderbilt.edu

Crit Care Nurs Clin N Am 29 (2017) 519–537
http://dx.doi.org/10.1016/j.cnc.2017.08.010
0899-5885/17/© 2017 Elsevier Inc. All rights reserved.

INTRODUCTION

Approximately 46.8 million individuals in 2015 were living with dementia worldwide, with a new case every 3.2 seconds.[1] In the United States, chronic pain is considered a "problem of epidemic proportions,"[2] affecting around 100 million adults.[3] Thus, the occurrence of pain and dementia increases with age,[4–6] presenting challenges for pain assessment in both long-term care (LTC) and adult critical care. Cognitively impaired individuals report pain less frequently and receive minimal[7] to no pain medication,[8] even when there is a known condition that causes pain, such as cancer.[7] Pain at rest in the intensive care unit is common in adult patients and contributes to complications.[9] Although multiple tools exist to help assess pain in dementia,[6,10,11] pain remains underassessed and inadequately treated.[8,12,13]

Behavioral and psychological symptoms of dementia (BPSD), such as agitation, may indicate pain in people with dementia.[14–16] Pain exacerbates agitation and may cause psychosis and delusions in dementia.[17] Medications, such as antipsychotics, are often overused and have significant adverse events in the dementia population.[18] Complementary and alternative medicine (CAM) may offer a less invasive, safer, and more gentle option to treat BPSD,[19–21] as well as pain,[19,20,22] and improve quality of life.[20,23,24] Reducing BPSD may also reduce the burden on the critical care nurse and support staff.[25] With opioid use becoming more scrutinized,[26] CAM therapies may help to decrease opioid use for pain.

CAM includes therapies such as aromatherapy, acupuncture, animal therapy, music, exercise, herbal medicine, massage, yoga,[23] therapeutic/healing touch,[24,27] tai chi, meditation, and dietary supplements.[28] CAM therapies have been used by nurses for many years,[29] and by many people over 65 years of age in the United States, Canada, United Kingdom, and Australia.[30] In a study of 32 countries across the globe, traditional, complementary, and alternative medicine ranges from 10% in Eastern Europe to more than 50% in Asia, with high treatment satisfaction rates of more than 80% in Europe, Asia, and the United States.[31] CAM has also been used in varying degrees in LTC for years.[19,20,30] Increased understanding and investigating appropriate use of CAM is also a national priority in the United States through the National Center for Complementary and Integrative Health,[32] formerly known as the National Center for Complementary and Alternative Medicine.

This paper reviews CAM therapies and their effectiveness when used in older adults with pain and dementia in LTC and to explore what CAM therapies used in LTC would feasibly transition to the critical care setting. To our knowledge, no literature review has been published to address this particular question. This review was guided by the authors' beliefs that, because the popularity of CAM will likely increase in LTC, critical care nurses receiving patients with dementia from LTC should question the communicative patient with dementia and their caregivers about current CAM use. This measure is especially important, because BPSD may increase with hospital admission, and discontinuing currently used CAM may exacerbate these symptoms and increase pain if CAM therapy is stopped abruptly.

SEARCH STRATEGY

PubMed and Google Scholar were searched for the terms: complementary, alternative, complementary alternative medicine, nursing home, residential care, LTC, dementia, Alzheimer's, and pain. These were used in multiple combinations with each other, and with and without AND, and with and without quotes. The terms pediatric, review, systematic, and book were used with the minus sign to reduce results of some searches on Google Scholar. Only results in English between the dates of 2002 to 2017 were used. Additional filters were added on PubMed for clinical trials and human trials only. Reference lists were reviewed for relevant citations. The Vanderbilt University Library was also searched for journals. Using the "contains" search option, the terms complementary and alternative, as well as dementia, were used individually to find relevant journals, such as *Journal of Complementary and Alternative Medicine*, *BMC Complementary and Alternative Medicine*, *Alternative and Complementary Therapies*, *Complementary Therapies in Clinical Practice*, *Complementary Therapies in Medicine*, *Evidence-based Complementary and Alternative Medicine*, *Journal of Evidence Based Complementary and Alternative Medicine*, *Journal of Traditional and Complementary Medicine*, and *Alzheimer's and Dementia*. Notably, owing to the lack of literature on CAM used to treat pain in dementia in LTC, we expanded our search for randomized, controlled trials to CAM use in patients with dementia.

Using this strategy, the final inclusion criteria for studies in this review were: (1) randomized controlled trial, (2) sample size of more than 10, (3) written in the English, (4) published between 2002 and 2017, (5) participant diagnosed with dementia, and (6) study performed in an LTC facility. A larger population size was initially preferred (n > 50); however, owing to limited results we determined that smaller sample sizes (N > 14) had to be included. Exclusion criteria were (1) articles not in English, (2) qualitative studies, (3) had a CAM therapy deemed less applicable to a critical care setting, or (4) did not meet inclusion criteria.

RESULTS

A total of 510 records were identified and screened, with 473 being excluded because they were not applicable to BPSD or interventions that could translate to inpatient care. The remaining 37 were evaluated in detail. Of these, 7 quantitative studies that best met inclusion criteria were included. **Tables 1–3** detail features of each study. For the 7 applicable studies, the setting and sample of each was in 1 or multiple LTC facilities, located across the globe in the United States, Canada, Japan, the United Kingdom, and 3 in Australia. There were 364 total randomized male and female participants aged 60 and older with dementia of various types across the reviewed studies. All but 2 studies had more than 50 participants, with sample sizes ranging from 14 to 94 **(Table 1)**.

Review results indicate there are multiple previous studies showing improvement in dementia symptoms[33,34] as well as reduction of pain[33–35] and stress[33,35] with aromatherapy, and 4 of the 7 studies included aromatherapy as an intervention.[35–38] Intervention variables also mostly involved touch in the form of foot[39] or hand massage,[36,37] reflexology,[40] therapeutic touch,[21] and dermally applied aromatherapy.[35–38] Outcome variables were primarily BPSD (especially agitation),[21,35–38] but also pain,[40] changes in mood and communication,[37] and physiologic stress responses (blood pressure, heart rate, salivary α-amylase)[39,40] (see **Table 2**).

DISCUSSION

In contrast with previous studies, often with less rigorous designs, findings demonstrated no improvement with aromatherapy in any of the studies. However, there is a trend where touch, interaction, and the presence of another human being improved BPSD, that other studies reflect as well.[27,41] Reflexology, in particular, did show a reduction in pain and α-amylase, a marker of stress,[40] and although regular foot

Table 1
Study characteristics

Author/Year/Country	Purpose/Aim	Design	Sample/Setting	Inclusion/Exclusion Criteria
Hodgson and Andersen,[40] 2008, United States	To assess the efficacy of reflexology in treating pain, distress, and negative affect in a population suffering from mild-to-moderate dementia	Quantitative: Randomized, experimental, repeated-measures, crossover design over 8 wk	N = 21 Residents of a 324-bed nursing home in suburban Philadelphia	Inclusion: Residents of the nursing home for ≥6 mo, 75 y of age or older, dementia diagnosis probable, able and willing to participate for the entire study, signed consent or verbal assent. Exclusion: Based on reflexology literature: history of deep vein thrombosis, epilepsy, bile or kidney stones, pacemaker, fever, open foot wounds, foot fractures. Also, recent hospitalization (<1 mo) preceding or during the study, and recent onset or discontinuation (<2 wk) of physiotherapy that included massage.
Fu et al,[36] 2013, Australia	To examine the ability of 3% lavender oil spray aromatherapy to treat disruptive behaviors in dementia populations living in LTC facilities	Quantitative: Single-blinded, randomized controlled trial of 3 groups with a placebo, over 6 wk	N = 67 Residents from 3 LTC facilities in Brisbane	Inclusion: To avoid persons with early onset dementia, aged 60 or over; in a nursing home for ≥3 mo to avoid potential effects from transition to the nursing home; MMSE score of 24 out of 30 or less; features of AD according to APA DSM-IV-TR; in the past 3 mo documented history of ≥2 wk of agitation or aggression (consecutively or 14 single days); documented physical and/or chemical restraint for agitation and aggression (including PRN medication); consent for participation from resident's family or health-attorney; no known allergic reaction to lavender oil; no recent skin tears, lacerations, bruises, or redness and swelling that might interfere with hand massage. Exclusion: Diagnosis of schizophrenia or mental retardation to avoid the complication of dual diagnoses impacting treatment effect; expectation of transfer to another facility within the next 3 mo.

Study	Purpose	Design	Sample	Criteria
Hawranik et al,[21] 2008, Canada	Compared usual care with therapeutic touch therapy (including simulated) in patients with AD. Also to improve limitations of previous studies	Quantitative: Randomized, multiple time series, blinded, 3-group experimental design	N = 51 Permanent residents from the personal care and special needs units of a LTC facility with AD (no city given)	Inclusion: Diagnosis of senile dementia of the AD type; a score of 23 or less on the MMSE; ≥65 y old; consistent agitated behavior during the past month or a history of agitated behavior; 2 or more months residence on the current unit; and the absence of an acute illness during the study. Exclusion: If the resident refused verbal consent (this was not specifically stated as exclusion criteria).
O'Connor et al,[35] 2013, Australia	To determine effectiveness of lavender (Lavandula angustifolia) oil as a treatment for objectively assessed agitation in patients with dementia. Also to help remedy methodologic shortcomings of previous studies	Quantitative: Randomized, single-blind cross-over trial	N = 64 Residents with frequent physically agitated behaviors from 8 specialist psychogeriatric nursing homes and 3 private nursing homes in Melbourne, between 2009 and 2011	Inclusion: Clinical Dementia Rating scale rating of mild or worse; physically agitated behavior requiring staff intervention occurring at least several times each day during daylight hours outside of nursing care; an assessment by the nursing staff, visiting medical practitioner, and/or psychiatrist that the behavior was not owing primarily to pain, physical illness, depression or psychosis; 3 or more months of residence in the facility; and consent of participation by the next of kin or guardian. Exclusion: An acute, life-threatening illness; a variable psychotropic medication use; and a medical condition that prohibited topical oil use.
Moyle et al,[39] 2014, Australia	To determine if foot massage will decrease physiologic stress in people with dementia	Quantitative: Randomized controlled trial with within-subjects, crossover design	N = 53 Residents from 5 LTC settings, located in South-East Queensland	Inclusion: An age of 65 y or older; 2 mo or more permanent residence in the facility; diagnosis of dementia, or met the criteria for probable AD; MMSE score < 18; PAS score >3 during each day over a period of 1 wk; 2 feet; appropriate informed consent. Exclusion: Artificial legs.

(continued on next page)

Table 1
(continued)

Author/Year/Country	Purpose/Aim	Design	Sample/Setting	Inclusion/Exclusion Criteria
Yoshiyama et al,[37] 2015, Japan	To determine the effectiveness and safety of clinical aromatherapy and hand massage in people with dementia	Quantitative: Randomized, single-blind crossover pilot study. Qualitative: Observation records were collected	N = 14 Residents from a nursing home in Nara	Inclusion: Nursing home residents; ≥65 y of age; dementia diagnosed by the ICD- 10; mild-to-moderate dementia (score of 10–26 on the MMSE); score of III on the Independence Degree of Daily Living for the Demented Elderly scale; negative reaction on a patch test with jojoba oil and D&H oil; and consent for participation from patients and their families. Exclusion: Any acute physical illness.
Burns et al,[38] 2011, UK	Compared the use of Melissa oil (*M officinalis*) aromatherapy with donepezil in treating BPSD in patients with AD	Quantitative: Double-blind, placebo-controlled randomized trial	N = 94 Residents from 3 LTC facilities in Manchester, London, and Southampton	Inclusion: Four weeks or more of agitation; ≥60 y of age; CMAI score of 139; NHS continuing care facility or nursing home resident; clinical dementia rating of 3; no psychotropic medication use (antipsychotics and/or cholinesterase inhibitors) for a minimum of 2 wk; written informed consent from patients when appropriate, and written assent was obtained from all caregivers. Exclusion: Known sensitivity to cholinesterase drugs; a disability preventing completing the study; severe, unstable, or poorly controlled medical conditions (particularly uncontrolled epilepsy, severe or unstable cardiovascular disease, severe asthma or severe chronic obstructive airways disease) or a history of stroke.

Abbreviations: AD, Alzheimer disease; APA, American Psychiatric Association; BPSD, behavioral and psychological symptoms; CMAI, Cohen Mansfield Agitation Inventory; D&H, Delight and Harmony oil; DSM-IV-TR, *Diagnostic and Statistical Manual, 4th edition, Text Revision*; ICD, *International Classification of Diseases*; LTC, long-term care; MMSE, Mini-Mental Status Examination; NHS, National Health Service; PAS, Psychogeriatric Assessment Scales.

massage in another study did not show much difference outside of a larger reduction in blood pressure, the researchers noted that the presence of another person was beneficial to all groups.[39] Therapeutic touch decreased wandering and pacing, adding support for touch and presence being an important factor; however, the sham therapeutic touch did not demonstrate this.[21] Surprisingly, as each of these studies showed benefit from touch and presence, which intuitively makes sense, the study on hand massage with and without aromatherapy made no statistically significant difference on agitation.[36] Had there been a qualitative component to that study, it would be interesting to see if it showed other improvements.

The essential oil Melissa was not superior to placebo, but the placebo revealed that touch and interaction helped, adding to the trend.[38] High-strength lavender oil was found to be no better than control,[35] as was Delight and Harmony oil blend with hand massage; however, the investigators did show safety as well as positive experiences of participants.[37] See **Table 2** for more details. Overall, the results offered evidence for human presence and interaction as well as touch reducing BPSD, stress, and pain.

External essential oil or aromatherapy use has demonstrated favorable results in the past for patients, reduced caregiver distress,[42] as well as reduced stress in nurses and staff in critical care settings.[43] Despite the included randomized controlled trials showing no difference from placebo, the studies showed safety and tolerability for external use. Individuals with dementia often have impaired olfactory function,[34,36] which may explain in part the negative results of the aromatherapy studies. Also, there are anecdotal reports that too high of a dose of lavender essential oil can be stimulating,[44] and could therefore negate any relaxing properties, or even increase agitation. This finding could explain the differing results from earlier studies and the O'Connor and colleagues[35] study, because they used the strongest concentration per solution they could apply to the skin. Another issue with aromatherapy trials is that there are no standardized or ideal doses or concentrations recognized,[35] and most studies vary widely in their demographics, methods, outcomes, and so on. This lack of standardization is problematic, because studies may miss potential benefits owing to improper strength, timing, or frequency, and cross-study comparisons are difficult. Other limitations of each study are listed in **Table 3**, including small sample sizes, questions of generalizability to larger populations, compliance with the intervention, subjective judgments by staff about scoring, and concomitant medication use by participants that might interfere with results.

An additional article was not included in the review because it was a debate paper that showed laughter and humor as a CAM treatment for dementia.[23] Takeda[23] argues that laughter is worth trying on an individualized basis, and explains the compelling physiologic basis for this option. Additional articles on essential oil use in BPSD[42,45,46] and cognitive function[47,48] showed positive results, but were not reviewed, because they did not meet inclusion criteria owing to study type, sample size, or applicability of the outcome variables. Other reviews that might be helpful resources for additional CAM options are Bauer and colleagues'[22] CAM in chronic pain and Wardell and Weymouth's review on healing touch,[27] as well as a large review showing that music therapy and behavioral management techniques were effective for BPSD.[49] Traditional Chinese Medicine was not included in this review, but is widely used in Asia[50,51] and has several compelling studies looking at cognitive function in dementia,[52,53] as well as on BPSD and activities of daily living in patients with dementia.[54] Abruptly stopping these, or other, CAM therapies upon patient admission may have unfavorable results.

Table 2
Description of variables and study results

Author/Year/Country	Intervention	Outcome Variables	Descriptive Results
Hodgson and Andersen,[40] 2008, United States	Treatment of 4 wk of weekly reflexology treatments followed by 4 wk of a control condition of friendly visits, or vice versa	Reduction of physiologic distress as measured by salivary α-amylase; secondary outcome was observed pain	A statistically significant decrease in observed pain ($P = .031$) and salivary α-amylase ($P = .049$) was found along with an improvement in sadness that nearly reached statistical significance ($P = .069$). No adverse events were reported.
Fu et al,[36] 2013, Australia	Treatment with aromatherapy spray (3% lavender oil) and hand massage or hand massage or placebo water spray twice daily for 6 wk	Agitation, aggression, and cognitive function via MMSE scores	No significant effect for the reduction of aggression or agitation was found for any of the study's measures.
Hawranik et al,[21] 2008, Canada	Treatment with therapeutic touch, sham (simulated), or usual care	Three forms of disruptive behavior: physical aggression, physical nonaggression, and verbal agitation	Physically nonaggressive behaviors were significantly reduced in the therapeutic touch group ($P<.05$), but no significant differences were found for a reduction in physical aggression or verbal agitation in all groups. All groups showed improvement overall, but the greatest improvements were in the therapeutic touch and sham therapeutic touch groups.
O'Connor et al,[35] 2013, Australia	Treatment with dermally applied, neurophysiologically active, high- purity 30% lavender oil in jojoba oil, or just jojoba oil	Physically agitated behaviors or affect improvement	No significant findings were reported for the efficacy of dermally applied lavender oil in treating agitation or improving affect in this sample.

Study	Intervention	Outcome measures	Results
Moyle et al,[39] 2014, Australia	Treatment with foot massage vs quiet presence	Physiologic stress response (eg, blood pressure and heart rate)	Foot massage as a therapy had no significant effect between groups, but both groups experienced an overall reduction in blood pressure with the foot massage group having a greater drop in systolic blood pressure than the control. A significant effect for the presence of human interaction was supported by a reduction in blood pressure and heart rate and remains a seemingly valid option in reducing agitation and distress in those with dementia.
Yoshiyama et al,[37] 2015, Japan	Treatment with clinical aromatherapy with D&H oil (blend of *Citrus aurantium* leaf, *Cymbopogon martini, Picea mariana, Lavandula angustifolia, Rosa damascena, Citrus paradisi,* and *M officinalis*) massaged gently on one hand and then the other in the following order: forearm, wrist, palm, fingers, and back of the hand, vs control therapy with jojoba oil administered in the same way	Effects on BPSD of dementia or ADL Changes in mood, behavior, communication (verbal and nonverbal)	Quantitative: No significant changes were found in agitation (assessed by CMAI), BPSD (assessed by NPI-Q), and ADLs (assessed by FIM). Additionally, there were no longitudinal improvements over 4 wk for any measure. No adverse effects were found. Qualitative: Participants had positive experiences during and after therapy, such as improved mood and sleep, and some experienced increases in both verbal and nonverbal communication.
Burns et al,[38] 2011, UK	Treatment with placebo medication and active aromatherapy (Melissa oil); active medication (donepezil) and placebo aromatherapy; or placebo of both	Effects on agitation	No evidence in support of the validity of Melissa as a treatment for agitation in AD when compared with donepezil and placebo was found. All groups, including placebo, experienced significant reduction in agitation levels after 12 wk, providing evidence for a nonspecific benefit of simple human interaction and touch in treating agitation. Adverse events for Melissa were the same as placebo.

Abbreviations: AD, Alzheimer disease; ADL, activities of daily living; BPSD, behavioral and psychological symptoms; CMAI, Cohen Mansfield Agitation Inventory; D&H, Delight and Harmony oil; FIM, Functional Independence Measure; MMSE, Mini-Mental Status Examination; NHS, National Health Service; NPI-Q, Neuropsychiatric Inventory–Questionnaire.

Table 3
Critique of research

Author/Year/Country	Threats and Biases	Limitations	Notes
Hodgson and Andersen,[40] 2008, United States	External validity: Generalizability/selection -small sample size that was homogeneous (all were white, female, Jewish, and in a nursing home, and 80% had Medicaid)	Although larger than many studies on this topic, the sample size limited the ability to analyze potential interactions of affect and α-amylase, and the sample was not randomly selected. The friendly visit portion of the control condition could have been stressful if the participant felt they had to put in effort to have a conversation, although this was not required, and it seems that this interaction was positive overall.	α-Amylase has been shown to be a valid physiologic measure for examining changes in affect and pain, so it is important to further examine the actions by which reflexology interacts with the sympathetic nervous system. A single reflexologist provided all treatment. Welden and Yesavage's progressive relaxation exercise was used before intervention and control Instruments: MMSE, CNPI, AARS, FAST
Fu et al,[36] 2013, Australia	External validity: Generalizability/selection – limited by sample size Internal validity: Performance bias possible – single blinded; participants not blinded (because of cognitive impairment) Instrumentation – despite training in CMAI, Participant behaviors were subjectively reported by staff Selective reporting bias – MMSE scores not reported (however, this was not their objective)	Olfactory functioning was not assessed in this population known to have potential olfactory deficits. Aromatherapy was given adjunctively with standard care practices and routine medications that might allow for the presence of unknown interactions. Because no standardized or ideal doses, concentrations, or forms of essential oils are recognized studies may miss potential benefits owing to improper strength, timing, frequency, or delivery method.	Trial registration ACTRN12612000917831; ethical and IRB approval obtained from the University Human Research Ethics Committee and the management of each aged care facility Instrumentation bias - issue reduced by inclusion of caregiver panel that rated behaviors as well Instruments: CMAI-SF, MMSE

Hawranik et al,[21] 2008, Canada	External validity: Generalizability/selection – limited by sample size Internal validity: Instrumentation – Research staff did not directly observe behaviors before or after intervention	The proposed underlying mechanism of this modality is questionable. Did not explore the mechanisms of therapeutic touch or its interactions with behaviors often exhibited in dementias of various types and severities or with longitudinal aspects such as time of day or year. The authors assert that because the patient is not actually touched, the benefits of touch should not be attributed to Therapeutic Touch's effects; however, the presence, attention, and warmth of a hand close to the body may still carry similar influences the way touch might. The behaviors tracked were selected from those that ≥25% of the participants showed in the weeks leading up to the study, resulting in 3 categories that might not include all relevant behaviors. The reported number of participants to achieve statistical power was not obtained, and the presence of 3 groups indicates possible lack of sufficient data points. Therapeutic touch intervention was implemented in the evening and results were measured within 2 h, but participants potentially experienced fewer behavioral symptoms because of the time of day, although the presence of the sundowning phenomenon is noted. Authors note staff may have grown tired of reporting symptoms and may have recorded fewer of them, and there was vacation staff who did not know the residents as well (and possibly less staff than usual).	Ethical approval was obtained to ensure that no coercion of participants occurred and that confidentiality and anonymity were maintained All Therapeutic Touch providers were also registered nurses Instruments: CMAI, MMSE

(continued on next page)

Table 3
(continued)

Author/Year/Country	Threats and Biases	Limitations	Notes
O'Connor et al,[35] 2013, Australia	Internal validity: Selective reporting bias - data not reported separately for each phase of trial Performance bias possible – single blinded; participants not blinded (because of cognitive impairment); efficacy of nose clips used is questionable	Because no standardized or ideal doses, concentrations, or forms of essential oils are recognized studies may miss potential benefits owing to improper strength, timing, frequency, or delivery method. Dose of lavender was much higher than other studies; potential for unknown or stimulating effects. Medication use in this sample might affect results; however, efforts were made not to alter psychotropic medications.	Registered with the Australian and New Zealand Clinical Trials Registry (ACTRN 1260900569202), and approved by all relevant committees including the Monash University Human Research Ethics Committee The study was funded by the National Health and Medical Research Council (Grant #545843) and the Dementia Collaborative Research Center administered through the University of New South Wales. "Neither funding body, nor the supplier of materials, played any part in analyzing data and preparing this report." Authors noted: "Future researchers should consider measuring plasma levels of linalool and linalyl acetate as a check on absorption, and optimal dosing regimens and formulations have yet to be established"; no attempt was made to distinguish between types of dementia. Instruments: CMAI, MMSE, Philadelphia Geriatric Center Affect Rating Scale

Study			
Moyle et al,[39] 2014, Australia	Internal validity: Instrumentation – BP and HR measurements might be inaccurate in some cases where the participant's arm was lower than recommended by the equipment's manufacturer. Data attrition – occurred when participants refused to have BP or HR taken (0.6% missing data in the study). Selective reporting bias – MMSE scores not reported (however, this was not their objective).	Medication use, because it was not altered in this sample, might affect results.	Registered with the Australian and New Zealand Trials Registry (ACTRN 1262000658819) and was granted ethical approval by the University Human Research Ethics Committee. Funding for the conduct of the study came from the National Health and Medical Research Council (NHMRC Project grant: 597415). The authors note: a future study might review medication and its influence on physiologic measures; this intervention may be useful in reducing hypertension, which is acknowledged to have an influence on the progression of dementia. Took measures to avoid autonomic dysfunction issues that could be present in some forms of dementia Instruments: CMAI, MMSE
Yoshiyama et al,[37] 2015, Japan	External validity: Generalizability/selection – small sample size (only 14) and only elderly females Internal validity: Selection – small sample size	Researchers could be influenced by single-blind crossover from initial pilot study. Qualitative analysis did not report the complete process and should be addressed in follow-up so reliability and validity statistics are obtained. Because no standardized or ideal doses, concentrations, or forms of essential oils are recognized studies may miss potential benefits owing to improper strength, timing, frequency, or delivery method. Effective measurement of changes in BPSD and ADLs might not have been achieved in a small timeframe of 4 wk. Study methods should be compared with alternative treatments to strengthen confidence in efficacy.	Approved by Tenri Health Care University Human Research Ethics Committee and the management of the facility. Instruments: CMAI, NPI-Q, Cornell Scale for Depression in Dementia, Functional Independent Measure.

(continued on next page)

Table 3
(continued)

Author/Year/Country	Threats and Biases	Limitations	Notes
Burns et al,[38] 2011, UK	Internal validity: Attrition bias possible – 20 participants lost, but remainder still larger than most studies of this nature. Data attrition bias – noted only an estimated 50% compliance rate in using the interventions	Because no standardized or ideal doses, concentrations, or forms of essential oils are recognized studies may miss potential benefits owing to improper strength, timing, frequency, or delivery method. Compliance rate was only estimated at 50% and only assessed by how full the returned bottles were, which could show a significant flaw. There was a greater chance of false-positive findings, acknowledged by the authors, from multiple testing for secondary outcomes. As such, caution is needed with interpreting results.	Registered with the European trials agency (EudraCT No. 2005–003269–17) and was approved by the ethics committee (reference: 05/Q1407/213), the MHRA (CTA No. 23,148/0001/001–0001). Melissa oil was used instead of lavender because of the broader range of receptors upon which it acts. Numerous adverse events were reported and included combinations of donepezil, Melissa oil, and placebo, with Melissa and placebo having the same adverse events at 2 each. All 3 groups showed benefit, the authors feel from hand massage as noted in the results section. Instruments: PAS, NPI, Barthel scale of ADLs, Blau QOL scale

Abbreviations: AARS, Apparent Affect Rating Scale; ADL, activities of daily living; BP, blood pressure; BPSD, behavioral and psychological symptoms of dementia; CMAI, Cohen Mansfield Agitation Inventory; CNPI, Checklist of Nonverbal Pain Indicators; FAST, Functional Assessment Staging; IRN, institutional review board; MMSE, Mini-Mental Status Examination; NPI, Neuropsychiatric Inventory; PAS, Psychogeriatric Assessment Scales; QOL, quality of life.

LIMITATIONS AND STRENGTHS

Limitations of this review include the potential for study inclusion selection bias. Although the primary author followed the inclusion and exclusion criteria outlined, including other databases and a wider date range may have yielded additional studies meeting criteria. Randomized controlled trials are considered among the most rigorous findings owing to reduced risk of bias; however, owing to the limited number of randomized controlled trials available for the current review, a more detailed quality assessment of each randomized controlled trial was not performed outside of what is shown in **Tables 1–3**. Also, valuable information may have been found from other studies types, such as qualitative and nonrandomized studies. In addition, several articles were found during this review that had promising titles, and sometimes translated abstracts, but the full text was written in different languages such as German, Chinese, and Japanese, and could not be read. In particular, Traditional Chinese Medicine and other CAM therapies that are more traditionally found in Asian countries may have favorable evidence and research that is not accessible owing to language barriers. More translated research findings could improve our understating of effective CAM options and use.

Despite these limitations, there are numerous strengths in the current review. First, only randomized controlled trials were included in this review. Second, the studies included represented a variety of countries. Third, 5 of the 7 randomized controlled trials have sample sizes of more than 50 participants, indicating a reasonable amount of power to detect treatment effects. Fourth, the studies demonstrated that touch, presence of another person, and interaction with other persons seem to improve BPSD. Last, there seem to be conceptually safe CAM therapies used in LTC that, in theory, should transfer between LTC and critical care with little disruption in continuity of treatment.

We recommend that future research in this area should involve determining the dose, strength, and frequency of different essential oils, including absorbed levels of compounds in the plasma levels, something other authors mentioned as well.[35] Even though there is preliminary evidence in this area,[41,49] continued and further research into touch, interaction, and presence for people with dementia would be helpful, as well as comparing different types of touch (eg, reflexology showed more favorable results than did regular foot massage).

CONCLUSION AND RECOMMENDATIONS

Aromatherapy is gaining more popularity and studies show favorable experiences and attitudes from nurses, staff, and caregivers using them in dementia care,[33,42,55] as well as improved quality of life for those with dementia.[25] Despite mixed results in efficacy, aromatherapy is generally safe when used externally, is inexpensive, and is rated as pleasant for the staff and patients.[42,55] Conceptually, we believe this modality could be used in both LTC and critical care, even if only to facilitate more touch, interaction, and human presence with the patient, and create a more relaxing environment for patients and staff.

Based on the current review and limited empirical evidence, we recommend that all acute care hospitals receiving patients from LTC facilities screen for current CAM use in people with dementia through direct questions with both communicative individuals with dementia and their caregivers. Furthermore, we recommend that critical care nurses receiving and caring for patients with dementia who normally reside in LTC should further assess for the use of CAM in persons with dementia and not rely solely on a history and physical received on admission, especially because CAM therapies may not be a common part of intake assessments. Upon hospital admission, and when possible, patient care may be improved by continuing any CAM therapy currently used by the patient. The critical care nurse may also be able to add helpful CAM therapies that may transition back to the home or LTC setting, improving overall patient care. Modalities that can reduce stress and agitation, such as touch and massage, may also reduce pain, and vice versa.[17] An open mind and thoughtful consideration of CAM therapy's effectiveness contributes to the widening variety of safer options to help improve the quality of life of people with dementia.

REFERENCES

1. Alzheimer's Disease International. World Alzheimer report 2015: the global impact of dementia. 2015. Available at: https://www.alz.co.uk/research/WorldAlzheimer Report2015-sheet.pdf. Accessed January 14, 2017.

2. Pain: current understanding of assessment, management, and treatments. American Pain Society, NPC. 2005. Available at: http://americanpainsociety.org/uploads/education/npc.pdf. Accessed January 14, 2017.

3. Institute of Medicine. Relieving pain in America. The National Institutes of Health 2011. Available at: http://www.nationalacademies.org/hmd/~/media/Files/Report Files/2011/Relieving-Pain-in-America-A-Blueprint-for-Transforming-Prevention-Care-Education-Research/Pain Research 2011 Report Brief.pdf. Accessed January 14, 2017.

4. Monroe TB, Herr KA, Mion LC, et al. Ethical and legal issues in pain research in cognitively impaired older adults. Int J Nurs Stud 2013;50(9):1283–7.

5. Pain in people with dementia: a silent tragedy. Available at: http://www.carechartsuk.co.uk/wp-content/uploads/2014/03/See-Change-Think-PainNapp-Report.pdf. Accessed January 14, 2017.

6. Chang SO, Oh Y, Park EY, et al. Concept analysis of nurses' identification of pain in demented patients in a nursing home: development of a hybrid model. Pain Manag Nurs 2011;12(2):61–9.

7. Monroe TB, Misra SK, Habermann RC, et al. Pain reports and pain medication treatment in nursing home residents with and without dementia. Geriatr Gerontol Int 2014;14(3):541–8.

8. Monroe TB, Carter MA, Feldt KS, et al. Pain and hospice care in nursing home residents with dementia and terminal cancer. Geriatr Gerontol Int 2013;13(4):1018–25.

9. Garrett KM. Best practices for managing pain, sedation, and delirium in the mechanically ventilated patient. Crit Care Nurs Clin North Am 2016;28(4):437–50.

10. Monroe TB, Mion LC. Patients with advanced dementia: how do we know if they are in pain? Geriatr Nurs 2012;33(3):226–8.

11. Abbey J, Piller N, De Bellis A, et al. The Abbey pain scale: a 1-minute numerical indicator for people with end-stage dementia. Int J Palliat Nurs 2004;10(1):6–13.

12. Monroe TB, Gore JC, Chen LM, et al. Pain in people with Alzheimer disease: potential applications for psychophysical and neurophysiological research. J Geriatr Psychiatry Neurol 2012;25(4):240–55.

13. Monroe TB, Misra S, Habermann RC, et al. Specific physician orders improve pain detection and pain reports in nursing home residents: preliminary data. Pain Manag Nurs 2015;16(5):770–80.

14. Monroe T, Carter M, Feldt K, et al. Assessing advanced cancer pain in older adults with dementia at the end-of-life. J Adv Nurs 2012;68(9):2070–8.

15. Paulson CM, Monroe T, Mion LC. Pain assessment in hospitalized older adults with dementia and delirium. J Gerontol Nurs 2014;40(6):10–5.

16. Burns M, McIlfatrick S. Nurses' knowledge and attitudes towards pain assessment for people with dementia in a nursing home setting. Int J Palliat Nurs 2015;21(10):479–87.

17. Habiger TF, Flo E, Achterberg WP, et al. The interactive relationship between pain, psychosis, and agitation in people with dementia: results from a cluster-randomised clinical trial. Behav Neurol 2016;2016:7036415.

18. Morley JE. Managing persons with dementia in the nursing home: high touch trumps high tech. J Am Med Dir Assoc 2008;9(3):139–46.

19. Allcock N, McGarry J, Elkan R. Management of pain in older people within the nursing home: a preliminary study. Health Soc Care Community 2002;10(6):464–71.

20. Webber GR. Complementary therapies in dementia care: which therapies are used in South Australian Nursing Homes? Counterpoints 2003;3(1):61–71.

21. Hawranik P, Johnston P, Deatrich J. Therapeutic touch and agitation in individuals with Alzheimer's disease. West J Nurs Res 2008;30(4):417–34.

22. Bauer BA, Tilburt JC, Sood A, et al. Complementary and alternative medicine therapies for chronic pain. Chin J Integr Med 2016;22(6):403–11.

23. Takeda M, Hashimoto R, Kudo T, et al. Laughter and humor as complementary and alternative medicines for dementia patients. BMC Complement Altern Med 2010;10:28.

24. Cai F-F, Zhang H. Effect of therapeutic touch on agitated behavior in elderly patients with dementia: a review. Int J Nurs Sci 2015;2:324–8.

25. Fung JK, Tsang HW, Chung RC. A systematic review of the use of aromatherapy in treatment of behavioral problems in dementia. Geriatr Gerontol Int 2012;12(3):372–82.

26. Hwang CS, Chang HY, Alexander GC. Impact of abuse-deterrent OxyContin on prescription opioid utilization. Pharmacoepidemiol Drug Saf 2015;24(2):197–204.

27. Wardell DW, Weymouth KF. Review of studies of healing touch. J Nurs Scholarsh 2004;36(2):147–54.

28. Kraft K. Complementary/alternative medicine in the context of prevention of disease and maintenance of health. Prev Med 2009;49(2–3):88–92.

29. Snyder M, Wieland J. Complementary and alternative therapies: what is their place in the management of chronic pain? Nurs Clin North Am 2003;38(3):495–508.

30. Bauer M, Rayner JA. Use of complementary and alternative medicine in residential aged care. J Altern Complement Med 2012;18(11):989–93.

31. Peltzer K, Pengpid S. Prevalence and determinants of traditional, complementary and alternative medicine provider use among adults from 32 countries. Chin J Integr Med 2016. [Epub ahead of print].

32. The National Center for Complementary and Integrative Health (NCCIH) - at a glance. Available at: https://nccih.nih.gov/about/ataglance. Accessed March 24, 2017.

33. Buckle J. Clinical aromatherapy. 2nd edition. Edinburgh (Scotland): Churchill Livingstone; 2003.

34. Snow LA, Hovanec L, Brandt J. A controlled trial of aromatherapy for agitation in nursing home patients with dementia. J Altern Complement Med 2004;10(3):431–7.

35. O'Connor DW, Eppingstall B, Taffe J, et al. A randomized, controlled cross-over trial of dermally-applied lavender (Lavandula angustifolia) oil as a treatment of agitated behaviour in dementia. BMC Complement Altern Med 2013;13:315.

36. Fu CY, Moyle W, Cooke M. A randomised controlled trial of the use of aromatherapy and hand massage to reduce disruptive behaviour in people with dementia. BMC Complement Altern Med 2013;13:165.

37. Yoshiyama K, Arita H, Suzuki J. The effect of aroma hand massage therapy for people with dementia. J Altern Complement Med 2015;21(12):759–65.

38. Burns A, Perry E, Holmes C, et al. A double-blind placebo-controlled randomized trial of Melissa officinalis oil and donepezil for the treatment of agitation in Alzheimer's disease. Dement Geriatr Cogn Disord 2011;31(2):158–64.

39. Moyle W, Cooke ML, Beattie E, et al. Foot massage and physiological stress in people with dementia: a randomized controlled trial. J Altern Complement Med 2014;20(4):305–11.

40. Hodgson NA, Andersen S. The clinical efficacy of reflexology in nursing home residents with dementia. J Altern Complement Med 2008;14(3):269–75.

41. Kim EJ, Buschmann MT. The effect of expressive physical touch on patients with dementia. Int J Nurs Stud 1999;36(3):235–43.

42. Turten Kaymaz T, Ozdemir L. Effects of aromatherapy on agitation and related caregiver burden in patients with moderate to severe dementia: a pilot study. Geriatr Nurs 2017;38(3):231–7.

43. Johnson K, West T, Diana S, et al. Use of aromatherapy to promote a therapeutic nurse environment. Intensive Crit Care Nurs 2017;40:18–25.

44. Worwood VA. The fragrant pharmacy. New York: Bantam Books Ltd; 1992.

45. Smallwood J, Brown R, Coulter F, et al. Aromatherapy and behaviour disturbances in dementia: a randomized controlled trial. Int J Geriatr Psychiatry 2001;16(10):1010–3.

46. Holmes C, Hopkins V, Hensford C, et al. Lavender oil as a treatment for agitated behaviour in severe dementia: a placebo controlled study. Int J Geriatr Psychiatry 2002;17(4):305–8.

47. Jimbo D, Kimura Y, Taniguchi M, et al. Effect of aromatherapy on patients with Alzheimer's disease. Psychogeriatrics 2009;9(4):173–9.

48. Akhondzadeh S, Noroozian M, Mohammadi M, et al. Melissa officinalis extract in the treatment of patients with mild to moderate Alzheimer's disease: a double blind, randomised, placebo controlled trial. J Neurol Neurosurg Psychiatry 2003;74(7):863–6.

49. Abraha I, Rimland JM, Trotta FM, et al. Systematic review of systematic reviews of non-pharmacological interventions to treat behavioural disturbances in older patients with dementia. The SENATOR-OnTop series. BMJ Open 2017;7(3): e012759.

50. Chung VC, Ma PH, Lau CH, et al. Views on traditional Chinese medicine amongst Chinese population: a systematic review of qualitative and quantitative studies. Health Expect 2014;17(5):622–36.

51. Wong E, Lam JKM, Griffiths S, et al. Chinese medicine: its role and application in the institutionalised older people. J Clin Nurs 2009;19:1084–93.

52. Iwasaki K, Kobayashi S, Chimura Y, et al. A randomized, double-blind, placebo-controlled clinical trial of the Chinese herbal medicine "ba wei di huang wan" in the treatment of dementia. J Am Geriatr Soc 2004;52(9):1518–21.

53. Zeng L, Zou Y, Kong L, et al. Can Chinese herbal medicine adjunctive therapy improve outcomes of senile vascular dementia? systematic review with meta-analysis of clinical trials. Phytother Res 2015;29(12):1843–57.

54. Iwasaki K, Satoh-Nakagawa T, Maruyama M, et al. A randomized, observer-blind, controlled trial of the traditional Chinese medicine Yi-Gan San for improvement of behavioral and psychological symptoms and activities of daily living in dementia patients. J Clin Psychiatry 2005;66(2):248–52.
55. Johannessen B. Nurses experience of aromatherapy use with dementia patients experiencing disturbed sleep patterns. An action research project. Complement Ther Clin Pract 2013;19(4):209–13.

UNITED STATES POSTAL SERVICE® Statement of Ownership, Management, and Circulation (All Periodicals Publications Except Requester Publications)

1. Publication Title	2. Publication Number	3. Filing Date
CRITICAL CARE NURSING CLINICS OF NORTH AMERICA	006 – 273	9/18/17

4. Issue Frequency	5. Number of Issues Published Annually	6. Annual Subscription Price
MAR, JUN, SEP, DEC	4	$155.00

7. Complete Mailing Address of Known Office of Publication (Not printer) (Street, city, county, state, and ZIP+4®)

ELSEVIER INC.
230 Park Avenue, Suite 800
New York, NY 10169

Contact Person
STEPHEN R. BUSHING
Telephone (Include area code)
215-239-3688

8. Complete Mailing Address of Headquarters or General Business Office of Publisher (Not printer)

ELSEVIER INC.
230 Park Avenue, Suite 800
New York, NY 10169

9. Full Names and Complete Mailing Addresses of Publisher, Editor, and Managing Editor (Do not leave blank)

Publisher (Name and complete mailing address)

ADRIANNE BRIGIDO, ELSEVIER INC.
1600 JOHN F KENNEDY BLVD. SUITE 1800
PHILADELPHIA, PA 19103-2899

Editor (Name and complete mailing address)

KERRY HOLLAND, ELSEVIER INC.
1600 JOHN F KENNEDY BLVD SUITE 1800
PHILADELPHIA, PA 19103-2899

Managing Editor (Name and complete mailing address)

PATRICK MANLEY, ELSEVIER INC.
1600 JOHN F KENNEDY BLVD. SUITE 1800
PHILADELPHIA, PA 19103-2899

10. Owner (Do not leave blank. If the publication is owned by a corporation, give the name and address of the corporation immediately followed by the names and addresses of all stockholders owning or holding 1 percent or more of the total amount of stock. If not owned by a corporation, give the names and addresses of the individual owners. If owned by a partnership or other unincorporated firm, give its name and address as well as those of each individual owner. If the publication is published by a nonprofit organization, give its name and address.)

Full Name	Complete Mailing Address
WHOLLY OWNED SUBSIDIARY OF REED/ELSEVIER, US HOLDINGS	1600 JOHN F KENNEDY BLVD. SUITE 1800 PHILADELPHIA, PA 19103-2899

11. Known Bondholders, Mortgagees, and Other Security Holders Owning or Holding 1 Percent or More of Total Amount of Bonds, Mortgages, or Other Securities. If none, check box ▶ ☐ None

Full Name	Complete Mailing Address
N/A	

12. Tax Status (For completion by nonprofit organizations authorized to mail at nonprofit rates) (Check one)
The purpose, function, and nonprofit status of this organization and the exempt status for federal income tax purposes:
☒ Has Not Changed During Preceding 12 Months
☐ Has Changed During Preceding 12 Months (Publisher must submit explanation of change with this statement)

13. Publication Title	14. Issue Date for Circulation Data Below
CRITICAL CARE NURSING CLINICS OF NORTH AMERICA	JUNE 2017

PS Form 3526, July 2014 [Page 1 of 4 (see instructions page 4)] PSN: 7530-01-000-9631 PRIVACY NOTICE: See our privacy policy on www.usps.com.

15. Extent and Nature of Circulation		Average No. Copies Each Issue During Preceding 12 Months	No. Copies of Single Issue Published Nearest to Filing Date
a. Total Number of Copies (Net press run)		264	208
b. Paid Circulation (By Mail and Outside the Mail)	(1) Mailed Outside-County Paid Subscriptions Stated on PS Form 3541 (Include paid distribution above nominal rate, advertiser's proof copies, and exchange copies)	146	115
	(2) Mailed In-County Paid Subscriptions Stated on PS Form 3541 (Include paid distribution above nominal rate, advertiser's proof copies, and exchange copies)	0	0
	(3) Paid Distribution Outside the Mails Including Sales Through Dealers and Carriers, Street Vendors, Counter Sales, and Other Paid Distribution Outside USPS®	45	35
	(4) Paid Distribution by Other Classes of Mail Through the USPS (e.g. First-Class Mail®)	0	0
c. Total Paid Distribution (Sum of 15b (1), (2), (3), and (4))	▶	191	150
d. Free or Nominal Rate Distribution (By Mail and Outside the Mail)	(1) Free or Nominal Rate Outside-County Copies included on PS Form 3541	45	58
	(2) Free or Nominal Rate In-County Copies Included on PS Form 3541	0	0
	(3) Free or Nominal Rate Copies Mailed at Other Classes Through the USPS (e.g. First-Class Mail)	0	0
	(4) Free or Nominal Rate Distribution Outside the Mail (Carriers or other means)	0	0
e. Total Free or Nominal Rate Distribution (Sum of 15d (1), (2), (3) and (4))	▶	45	58
f. Total Distribution (Sum of 15c and 15e)	▶	236	208
g. Copies not Distributed (See Instructions to Publishers #4 (page #3))	▶	28	0
h. Total (Sum of 15f and g)	▶	264	208
i. Percent Paid (15c divided by 15f times 100)	▶	80.93%	72.12%

* If you are claiming electronic copies, go to line 16 on page 3. If you are not claiming electronic copies, skip to line 17 on page 3.

16. Electronic Copy Circulation		Average No. Copies Each Issue During Preceding 12 Months	No. Copies of Single Issue Published Nearest to Filing Date
a. Paid Electronic Copies	▶	0	0
b. Total Paid Print Copies (Line 15c) + Paid Electronic Copies (Line 16a)	▶	191	150
c. Total Print Distribution (Line 15f) + Paid Electronic Copies (Line 16a)	▶	236	208
d. Percent Paid (Both Print & Electronic Copies) (16b divided by 16c × 100)	▶	80.93%	72.12%

☒ I certify that 50% of all my distributed copies (electronic and print) are paid above a nominal price.

17. Publication of Statement of Ownership
☒ If the publication is a general publication, publication of this statement is required. Will be printed
in the DECEMBER 2017 issue of this publication. ☐ Publication not required.

18. Signature and Title of Editor, Publisher, Business Manager, or Owner

STEPHEN R. BUSHING – INVENTORY DISTRIBUTION CONTROL MANAGER

Date 9/18/17

I certify that all information furnished on this form is true and complete. I understand that anyone who furnishes false or misleading information on this form or who omits material or information requested on the form may be subject to criminal sanctions (including fines and imprisonment) and/or civil sanctions (including civil penalties).

PS Form 3526, July 2014 (Page 3 of 4) PRIVACY NOTICE: See our privacy policy on www.usps.com

Printed and bound by CPI Group (UK) Ltd, Croydon, CR0 4YY

07/10/2024

01040503-0009